Tracheostomy Tubes and Ventilator Dependence in Adults and Children

A Handbook for the Speech-Language Pathologist

Kelly VanDahm, M.S., CCC-SLP

and

Sally Sparks-Walsh, M.S., CCC-SLP

Foreword by Shawn E. Wright, M.D., FCCP

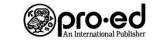

pro·ed
An International Publisher

8700 Shoal Creek Boulevard
Austin, Texas 78757-6897
800/897-3202   Fax 800/397-7633
www.proedinc.com

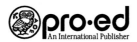

© 2002 by PRO-ED, Inc.
8700 Shoal Creek Boulevard
Austin, Texas 78757-6897
800/897-3202   Fax 800/397-7633
www.proedinc.com

Edited by Kirsteen E. Anderson
Illustrated by David Fischer
Cover design by Kelly Hume with illustration by David Fischer
Book design by Nancy Weaver

ISBN-13: 978-141640358-6
ISBN-10: 1-4164-0358-2

Previously published by Imaginart International, Inc. under ISBN 1-883315-58-1.

Printed in the United States of America

1 2   3   4   5   11 10   09   08   07

Acknowledgments

From Kelly

A special thank you to Joel, my husband, who throughout this process has provided me with loving encouragement and graciously held down the fort while putting up with the many demands on my time. You are a wonderful husband and a terrific dad! Thanks also to my family for emboldening me to continue to seek out new challenges. I would like to send many thanks to Kathy Drewitz, RN, Adrienne Lowe, CRT, and Sonya Postma, MS/CCC-SLP, for sharing their knowledge and support in the writing of this text. Thanks also to the awesome therapists of the speech, OT, PT and respiratory departments, and both the adult and pediatric nursing departments at Select Specialty Hospital in Phoenix, for teaching me that our patients' many successes come from strong interdisciplinary efforts and caring interventions.

From Sally

This undertaking certainly would not have been possible without the tremendous support and patience of my husband, Kevin. His thoughtfulness, understanding, support and encouragement made the process of writing this book bearable, and for that and much, much more, thank you and I love you. I would also like to thank my parents for their faith in me throughout the years, even though they never really knew what path I would end up taking. I would like to give special thanks to Richard Katz, Ph.D., CCC-SLP, whose confidence and guidance in my career and with this project have been considerable. Thanks to the speech-language pathologists, physicians, dietitians and respiratory therapists at the Carl T. Hayden VA Medical Center for their willingness to answer my never-ending lists of questions.

From Both of Us

We would like to thank all of the vendors for their cooperation and for providing photographs and product information. A special thank-you to Cindy and Ken Drolet at Imaginart and Kirsteen Anderson, our editor; we appreciate your patience with us and guidance through this process. Thanks also to David Fischer for providing the anatomical illustrations for this text.

Contents

Foreword xi

Introduction 1

1 Anatomical Overview of the Respiratory System 3
Components of the Respiratory System 3
Physiology of Respiration 9
Differences between Pediatric and Adult Anatomy 10

2 Issues Surrounding Patients with Complex Medical Needs 13
Medical Review 13
Medical History and Chart Review Form 16
Interdisciplinary Care Team 18
Understanding the Nature of the Diagnosis 20
Nutritional Status 21
Respiratory Status 24
Monitoring the Individual with Complex Medical Needs 24
Conclusion 28

3 Alternative Airways 31
Types of Intubation 31
Tracheotomy Procedure 34
Components of a Tracheostomy Tube 36
Components of an Endotracheal Tube 44
Types of Tracheostomy Tubes 45
Conclusion 51

4 Methods of Communication 53
Nonvocal Communication Options 55
Vocal Communication Options 57
Clinical Trials of a Speaking Valve 68
Speaking Valve Trial Flow Sheet 70
Using Speaking Valves with Infants and Children 73
Conclusion 77

5 Tracheostomy and Dysphagia 79
Phases of the Normal Swallow 79
Swallowing in Infants. 81
Influence of a Tracheostomy Tube on Swallowing 82
Issues Surrounding the Tracheostomy Cuff 84
Swallowing Assessment with a Tracheostomy Tube 87
Blue Dye Swallowing Assessment Tracking Form. 90
Strategies to Increase Swallowing Safety and Efficiency with a
  Tracheostomy Tube. 93
Conclusion 95

6 Mechanical Ventilation. 97
How a Ventilator Works. 97
Types of Ventilators 98
Ventilator Parameters and Terminology 100
Modes of Mechanical Ventilation 102
Ventilator Alarms 105
Vocal Communication with a Ventilator 110
In-Line Speaking Valve Trial Flow Sheet 114
Ventilators and Swallowing. 117
Ventilators and the Pediatric Population 119
Conclusion 121

7 Tracheostomy Care and Hygiene Issues. 123
Tracheostomy Care. 123
Speaking Valve Care 124
Maintaining a Patent Airway 124
Oral Hygiene. 127
Supplies to Keep Readily Available 128
Conclusion 131

**Appendix A: Clinical Values and Measurements Associated with Patient
  Monitoring and Care**. 133
Appendix B: Vendor List. 137
Appendix C: Patient and Family Education Pages 143

Glossary 153
Bibliography 165
Index. 171

Figures and Tables

Figures

1.1. Lateral view of the oral and nasal cavities. 4
1.2. Angles of bifurcation of the lungs, adult versus pediatric 5
1.3. Muscles of respiration and their levels of innervation 8
1.4. Five stages of respiration at the level of the alveoli 9
1.5. Differences between adult and pediatric oral and pharyngeal anatomy 10
1.6. Comparative diagrams of the adult and pediatric rib cage 11

2.1. Gastrointestinal system, showing placements of feeding tubes. 23
2.2. Pulse oximetry sensors 26

3.1. Lateral view of oral and nasal endotracheal intubation. 32
3.2. Manual resuscitation bag 33
3.3. Lateral view of tracheostomy tube, with cuff inflated 35
3.4. Portex percutaneous tracheotomy kit and percutaneous tracheostomy tube . 35
3.5. Fenestrated and unfenestrated outer cannulas 36
3.6. Fenestrated and unfenestrated inner cannulas 37
3.7. Standard 15 mm tracheostomy hub 38
3.8. Cuff and pilot balloon 39
3.9. Underinflated cuff. 40
3.10. Overinflated cuff 40
3.11. Bivona Fome-Cuf® tracheostomy tube. 41
3.12. Obturator. 42
3.13. Tracheostomy button 42
3.14. Tracheostomy collar or mask 43
3.15. Variety of heat-moisture exchange devices 43
3.16. Oral endotracheal tube and cuffless nasal endotracheal tube. 44
3.17. Cuffless fenestrated tracheostomy tube showing placement
     and components 45
3.18. Cuffless unfenestrated tracheostomy tube showing placement
     and components 46
3.19. Cuffed fenestrated tracheostomy tube showing placement
     and components 47
3.20. Cuffed unfenestrated tracheostomy tube showing placement
     and components 47

3.21. Granulation tissue partially obstructing the fenestrations of a tracheostomy tube 48

3.22. Jackson metal tracheostomy tube. 49

3.23. Shiley and Bivona neonate and pediatric tracheostomy tubes 50

4.1. Lateral view of oral endotracheal and tracheostomy tube placements 54

4.2. Four-cell augmentative communication device 56

4.3. Illustration of a talking tracheostomy tube system. 58

4.4. Bivona and Portex talking tracheostomy tubes 59

4.5. One-way speaking valve attached to the inner cannula hub 62

4.6. Shiley Phonate speaking valve 63

4.7. Montgomery speaking valve. 63

4.8. Variety of Passy-Muir speaking valves 64

4.9. Shikani-French speaking valve on a metal tracheostomy tube 65

4.10. Tucker valve 66

4.11. Clipped inner cannula with speaking valve attached 69

4.12. Child with PMV and infant with PMV. 75

5.1. Four stages swallowing 80

5.2. Overinflated cuff pressing into the esophagus and obstructing the passage of a bolus. 84

5.3. Tracheoesophageal fistula illustration and radiographic image 85

5.4. Aspirated material pooling in and around an underinflated tracheostomy cuff 86

5.5. Glucofilm® Test Strips for glucose testing 91

5.6. Swallowing workstation used for FEES® 93

6.1. In-line suctioning unit 98

6.2. Omni-Flex connector 98

6.3. Common brands of ventilators: PB 7200, Infant Star, and LTV 950. 99

6.4. PMV attached to ventilator tubing with Omni-flex 110

6.5. PMV attached in-line to a ventilator 113

6.6. Infant with PMV in-line with a ventilator 119

6.7. Child with PMV in-line with a ventilator 120

7.1. Tracheostomy cleaning kit 124

7.2. Sterile suctioning equipment 125

7.3. Sterile suctioning through a tracheostomy tube 125

7.4. Sterile suctioning through a nasal trumpet 126

7.5. In-line suctioning unit 126
7.6. Yankauer suction tip 127
7.7. Toothette oral swab attached to suctioning attachment port. 128
7.8. Personal protection equipment 129
7.9. Sterile examination gloves 129
7.10. Portable pulse oximeter 130

Tables

2.1. Criteria for assigning an Apgar score 15
4.1. Possible causes of and solutions to difficulty using a speaking valve 74
6.1. Comparison chart of modes of ventilation 106

Foreword

Increasingly, critically ill patients are surviving devastating illnesses that only a few years ago would certainly have resulted in death. Almost miraculous advances in medical and surgical intensive care have granted many seriously ill individuals a second chance at life. Unfortunately, this gift has not come without a price. Many patients pay a "survivor penalty" for their recovery. This penalty may include long-term care in a specialized facility, prolonged mechanical ventilation, and tracheostomy and feeding tube placement for ventilation and proper long-term nutrition. Thankfully, most of these patients eventually return home and recover to a point that is acceptable to themselves and their families.

The level of care required to achieve these results, however, is enormous. Successful recovery from critical illness is largely dependent upon expertly trained and dedicated professionals from many disciplines. Additionally, to effectively treat these patients with complex needs, caregivers in this era of medicine must possess a broad array of medical knowledge that may extend beyond the traditional boundaries of their original training. The challenge in taking care of the sick patient today is this: Miracles of medical care in the twenty-first century rest on the ability of medical professionals to grasp and put into practice the information, techniques and tools provided by rapidly appearing technological innovation.

Kelly VanDahm and Sally Sparks-Walsh have captured the essence of this challenge in *Tracheostomy Tubes and Ventilator Dependence in Adults and Children*. This book skillfully intertwines the practical with the cutting edge. Beginning with a review of anatomical and physiologic considerations important to the care of a patient who is very ill, VanDahm and Sparks-Walsh guide the practitioner through the landscape of airway management, vocal and nonvocal communication, swallowing assessment and mechanical ventilation. The handbook expertly and concisely covers topics often neglected in more esoteric texts on speech-language disorders in a format that allows the reader to access and utilize the information much more readily.

To paraphrase writer C. S. Lewis, we do not need to learn new things as much as we need to remember things which we already know. I thoroughly enjoyed the advance copy of *Tracheostomy Tubes and Ventilator Dependence in Adults and Children*. I have no doubt speech-language professionals who care for patients who are critically ill will recall the "pearls" from this book for a long time.

Shawn E. Wright, M.D.
Chairman, Division of Pulmonary Medicine
St Joseph's Hospital and Medical Center, Phoenix
Section Chief, Pulmonary Special Procedures
Arizona Pulmonary Specialists, Ltd.

Introduction

As humans, we all realize, and sometimes take for granted, that we have to breathe in order to live. But what happens when a traumatic injury, a degenerative disease, complications of surgery or the long-term effects of smoking take away a person's ability to breathe independently? How is breathing managed in this situation? And how do clinicians go about restoring communication and swallowing in such a patient?

Historically, most speech-language pathologists have typically worked with patients who were medically stable, had a single diagnosis and presented with clear speech and language deficits. The medical arena is changing and changing quickly. As medical treatment continues to improve and extends into new areas, clinicians will increasingly be faced with adults and children who have complex, and perhaps multiple, diagnoses. Such patients may be dependent on medical equipment and procedures that have altered their normal anatomical processes for maintaining intraventricular pressures, taking nutrition and even breathing. Moreover, as insurance reimbursement practices continue to change, patients are being sent home earlier and children with chronic medical needs are being mainstreamed into school systems. The responsibility for meeting their care needs is increasingly falling on the professionals who work with these individuals in their homes and schools.

Unfortunately, the curricula in most university degree programs have not been modified to address the evolving role of speech-language pathologists. Even though graduates have the basic knowledge and resources to treat patients with multiple, medically complex diagnoses, they are likely to need practical information about and clinical experience with this population. Now more than ever, speech-language pathologists need to take the initiative to expand their knowledge and expertise in medically related areas. In an effort to address these issues, we offer *Tracheostomy Tubes and Ventilator Dependence in Adults and Children*. This practical manual focuses on clinical issues of providing speech and language services to patients who are tracheotomized or ventilator-dependent. It provides information on clinical trials, diagrams, resources and vendor lists, as well as patient and family education pictures, reference norms, sample forms for documentation and an extensive glossary. We hope you will find this book to be a quick reference guide that will aid you in providing your adult and pediatric clients with the best possible care and helping them meet their communication and swallowing goals.

Chapter 1 reviews the anatomy and physiology of the respiratory system, providing the background necessary to understand subsequent chapters. Chapter 2 outlines the complex medical issues of tracheostomy and ventilator-dependent patients, including common diagnoses, medical interventions and patient monitoring procedures. Chapter 3 addresses reasons for intubation, different tracheotomy procedures, and the components and function of tracheostomy tubes. In chapter 4 the various communication options available to patients who are tracheotomized or ventilator-dependent are reviewed. Protocols for determining patients' candidacy for the various options and beginning clinical trials are discussed. Chapter 5 looks at how a tracheostomy tube affects the swallowing mechanism, as well as how to conduct swallowing assessments and treatment protocols with such patients. Basic information on how a mechanical ventilator works, how to troubleshoot ventilator alarms and how to address communication and swallowing with patients who are ventilator-dependent is covered in chapter 6. Chapter 7 addresses issues of tracheostoma hygiene and maintenance, as well as the supplies a clinician working with the tracheotomized population should have on hand. All chapters have discussions specific to infants and children when special protocols or considerations apply to these populations.

Chapter 1

Anatomical Overview of the Respiratory System

A good general understanding of the anatomy and physiology of respiration is necessary in order to design appropriate treatments for patients who are tracheotomized or ventilator-dependent, to identify and troubleshoot complications in treatment and to give an accurate prognosis of the outcome of treatment. It is also important to be aware of the differences between pediatric and adult anatomy. These issues will be discussed in this chapter.

Components of the Respiratory System

Respiration is regulated by the medulla oblongata and pons. Nerves at the cervical and thoracic levels of the spine innervate the muscles of inspiration, whereas expiration is largely passive. Several structures play important roles in the respiratory cycle, including the oral and nasal cavities, the larynx, the trachea and bronchi, and the lungs. The anatomy and physiology of these structures will be reviewed, with an emphasis on their role in respiration.

■ Anatomy and Physiology of the Oral and Nasal Cavities

The primary function of the oral and nasal cavities is to protect the airway and humidify inspired air (see figure 1.1, page 4). In the case of the nasal cavity, small mucus-covered hairs (cilia) covering the tissues provide its protection by trapping dust, pollen and other foreign bodies and moving them toward a means of expulsion (the nares or mouth). Moisture is maintained by the nasal turbinates. As air passes through the convoluted passages of the nasal turbinates, it draws moisture from the large surface area of the tissues and becomes humidified.

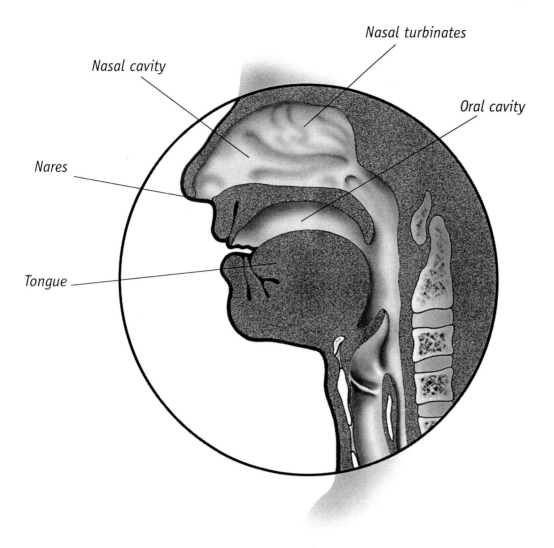

Figure 1.1. Lateral view of the oral and nasal cavities.

The structures within the oral cavity and the pharynx provide barriers to protect the larynx and the upper airway. If a foreign body is inadvertently inhaled, all these structures have the ability to obstruct the flow of the particle into the airway.

Anatomy and Physiology of the Larynx

The larynx has very important anatomical and physiological roles in respiration. Located within the thyroid cartilage, the larynx houses the vocal cords (also called vocal folds). In addition to their role in speech, the vocal cords have a protective function in that when closed completely they block the trachea, preventing foreign bodies from falling into the lungs. Coordinated movements of the larynx and vocal cords are vital to ensure the free flow of air during breathing, the protection of the lungs during swallowing and the production of phonation. For example, the vocal cords are abducted (opened) widely during quiet breathing, adducted (closed) slightly during exhalation, and adducted tightly prior to effortful coughing and throat clearing. During swallowing, the larynx moves upward and forward as the vocal cords close tightly, preventing food or liquid from entering the airway. As will be discussed in later chapters, the placement of an artificial airway significantly compromises the movement of the larynx and vocal cords, greatly increasing the risks of complications arising from aspiration.

■ Anatomy and Physiology of the Trachea and Bronchi

The trachea is the tube through which air moves into and out of the lungs. Starting below the larynx, it extends downward and ends at the point of bifurcation (splitting) where the left and right main bronchi (the main passages to the lungs) begin. The trachea is a cylindrical duct made up of between sixteen and twenty cartilaginous rings that maintain its patency (openness).

At the point of bifurcation of the trachea is the carina, the area which, when irritated, will elicit a cough reflex. The right main bronchus is shorter and wider and separates at a less acute angle than the left main bronchus (see figure 1.2). Because the angle of bifurcation is not as sharp on the right side, material is more likely to be aspirated into the right lower and middle lobes of the lung than into those on the left.

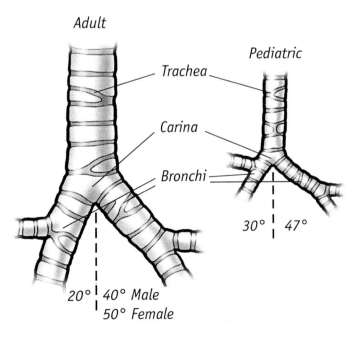

Figure 1.2. The angles of bifurcation of the lungs, adult versus pediatric.

Anatomy and Physiology of the Lungs

The left and right main bronchi lead from the trachea to the lungs. The lungs are bilateral cone-shaped structures located within the thorax (chest area). They are partially divided into lobes, with upper, middle and lower lobes on the right and only upper and lower lobes on the left.

Once the right and left main bronchi enter the lungs, there begins a complex series of divisions into smaller and smaller tubes called bronchioles. As the bronchioles continue to divide, they become bronchiole ducts and eventually terminate in alveoli. These tiny sacs contain a multitude of capillaries (tiny blood vessels) and are responsible for the diffusion, or exchange, of oxygen and carbon dioxide between the lungs and the bloodstream (discussed in more detail in the "Physiology of Respiration" section of this chapter). The distribution of the alveoli is an important factor in respiration, because the greatest and most efficient exchange of gases occurs where the greatest number of alveoli are. The distribution of alveoli is unequal, with the greatest number being located near the bases of the lungs. The alveoli are coated with a surfactant, a lipoprotein substance that prevents the alveoli from collapsing during exhalation and promotes the exchange of oxygen and carbon dioxide within the blood.

Musculature of Respiration

Below the lungs is the diaphragm, the principal muscle of respiration, which is responsible for 70 percent of the volume of inspired air. This thin, very strong sheet of muscular tissue separates the chest cavity from the abdominal cavity. When the diaphragm flattens, it increases the volume of the chest cavity and decreases the volume of the abdomen. This action begins the inspiratory cycle, during which air is drawn into the lungs.

The intercostal muscles couple the ribs together. During inspiration, the diaphragm and the intercostal muscles contract, causing the thorax and lungs to expand, and creating negative pressure (a partial vacuum) within the lungs that pulls air in. The passive release of the intercostal muscles during exhalation contributes to the recoil of the lungs, the return of the chest muscles to their resting state, and the exhalation of air out of the body.

The strap muscles, located in the neck, consist of the sternocleidomastoid and scalene muscles. These muscles, which assist the diaphragm and can increase the volume of a breath, are known as accessory muscles because they play a secondary role in inspiration. Together with the intercostals, the inspiratory accessory muscles can counterbalance a poorly functioning diaphragm to some degree. Individuals who have respiratory disease or difficulty often make such significant use of the strap muscles that these can be seen contracting during inspiration, a phenomenon sometimes referred to as "neck breathing."

In contrast to inspiration, exhalation is mostly passive (except during speech or singing); due to their elasticity, the lungs naturally recoil and return to their resting size and position. Because they are linked to the chest wall, however, they cannot contract completely, and a residual volume of air remains in the lungs, even with forced exhalation.

During controlled expiration, as with speech, the abdominal muscles, including the rectus abdominis, the internal and external obliques and the transversus abdominis are active. These muscles contract to compress the abdomen during expiration, which pushes against the diaphragm. Then they typically relax during inspiration. They are always active during speech breathing. In addition, many types of pulmonary disease damage the natural elasticity of the lungs, requiring the patient to use active exhalation to force air from the lungs. The process of exhalation becomes more difficult, and frequently air is "squandered" in the lungs. That is, because a larger residual volume of air remains in the lungs, less air can be inspired on the next breath, respiration is less efficient and the work of breathing intensifies.

Innervation of the Respiratory Muscles

Especially when working with individuals who have spinal cord injuries, it is important to recognize the different levels of innervation of the respiratory muscles in order to understand whether and how the injury may affect independent breathing (see figure 1.3, page 8). The diaphragm is innervated bilaterally by the phrenic nerve, which branches off from cervical spinal nerves C3 and C5. The thoracic spinal nerves T1 through T11 control the intercostal muscles. Cranial nerve XI and spinal nerves C2 through C8 innervate the strap muscles. Finally, the abdominal muscles are activated by thoracic and lumbar spinal nerves (T6–T12 and L1).

Regulatory Function of the Brain on Respiration

Ventilation, or the cyclical movement of air into and out of the lungs, is regulated by the respiratory center located in the medulla oblongata and the pons. The respiratory center functions to maintain stable gas exchange so carbon dioxide and oxygen levels remain balanced. A group of specialized nerve cells, called chemoreceptors, located in blood vessels such as the carotid artery, monitor the level of carbon dioxide in the blood. High levels of carbon dioxide—and hence inadequate levels of oxygen— trigger these chemoreceptors to send impulses to the respiratory center, which causes the rate of respiration to increase. Meanwhile, stretch receptors located in the smooth muscles of the airway monitor the expansion and deflation of the lungs and bronchi, sending impulses that help to regulate the respiratory cycle.

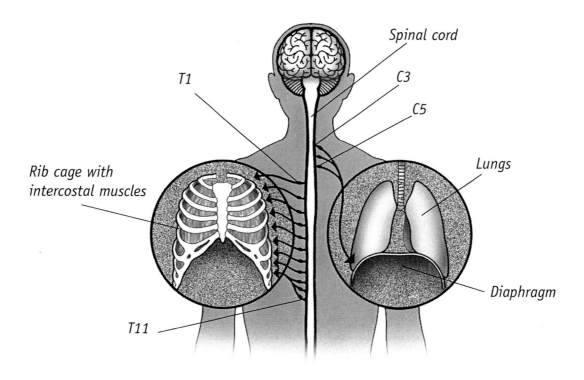

Figure 1.3. The muscles of respiration and their levels of innervation.

The deflation of the lungs activates the stretch receptors, which send information back to the respiratory center. The respiratory center then activates the muscles of inspiration by sending impulses via the spinal cord to the phrenic nerve, which controls the diaphragm, and to other spinal nerves that innervate the intercostal muscles. When the alveoli are fully inflated and have sufficient oxygen, the respiratory center sends an inhibition response that causes the muscles of inspiration to stop. Forced breathing and breathing to produce speech or singing are accomplished in a similar manner, though these types of breathing require controlled use of voluntary muscles for inspiration and expiration.

Physiology of Respiration

The normal course of respiration occurs in five stages. A disruption in any one of these stages lessens the oxygenation of the blood. (See figure 1.4 for diagrams of the stages.)

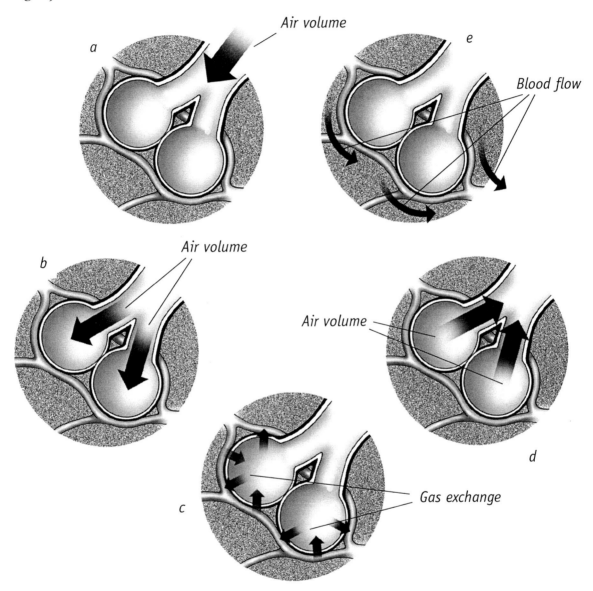

Figure 1.4. The five stages of respiration at the level of the alveoli: (a) ventilation; (b) distribution; (c) diffusion; (d) perfusion; and (e) circulation.

The process of respiration begins with ventilation, the movement of gases into and out of the lungs during inhalation and exhalation. During the distribution stage, the inhaled air travels to the alveoli, ideally those at the bases of the lungs, where gas exchange is most efficient. Since the greatest number of alveoli are present at the lung bases, this is where the greatest distribution occurs. Once the air reaches the alveoli, diffusion—the exchange of gases between the alveoli and bloodstream—occurs. Red blood cells give off waste carbon dioxide to the alveoli and pick up oxygen. The flow of blood through the pulmonary vessels, referred to as perfusion, must be adequate to accomplish this exchange, and obstruction of the pulmonary vessels can cause respiratory dysfunction. The process of circulation transports oxygenated blood to all the systems of the body and carries off waste carbon dioxide. The total volume of blood circulated throughout the body is called cardiac output.

Patients who are medically compromised may have poor functioning in any one or more of these stages. A tracheostomy tube and a ventilator may improve the processes of ventilation and distribution but cannot guarantee diffusion, perfusion or circulation.

Differences between
Pediatric and Adult Anatomy

Recognizing the differences between adult and pediatric anatomy is crucial. Although the components of the respiratory system and their functions are generally similar between adults and children, there are some very important anatomical differences that can affect the outcome of treatment. These differences are summarized here (see figure 1.5).

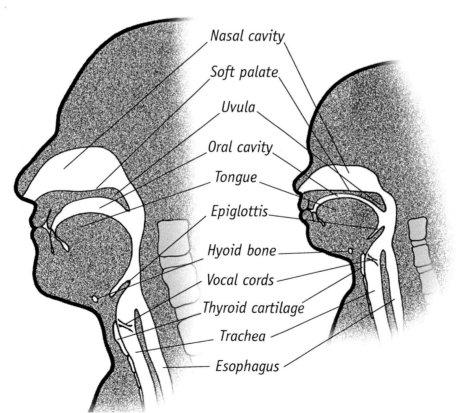

Figure 1.5. Differences between adult and pediatric oral and pharyngeal anatomy.

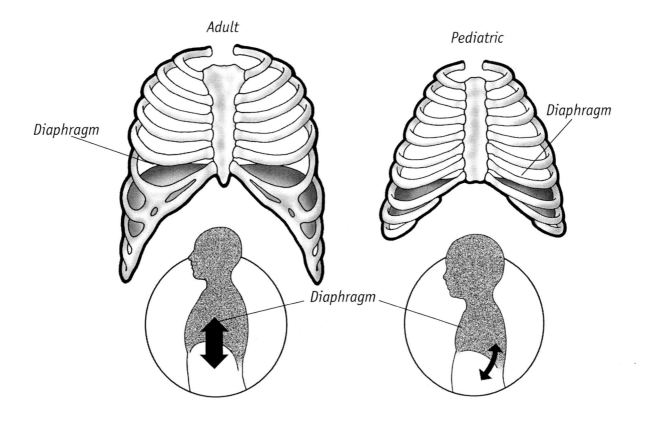

Adult

Pediatric

Diaphragm

Diaphragm

Diaphragm

Figure 1.6. Comparative diagrams of the adult and pediatric rib cage, showing diaphragmatic movement.

Soft palate. The size of the soft palate relative to the oral cavity is greater in an infant than in an adult. The large velum facilitates nasal breathing and interferes with mouth breathing in infants. By four to six months of age, the oral cavity has grown sufficiently to permit efficient mouth breathing, although many young children continue to prefer nasal breathing.

Uvula and epiglottis. The uvula, attached to this large soft palate, hangs much lower in infants than in adults. In fact, an infant's uvula actually contacts the top of the epiglottis, which is relatively more omega-shaped. The meeting of the uvula and the epiglottis facilitates the infant swallow while allowing nasal breathing to continue until the moment of the swallow itself.

Larynx/vocal cords. The location of the larynx is approximately two to three cervical vertebrae higher and is more anterior in infants and children than in adults.

Trachea. Because an infant's or child's tracheal diameter is much smaller than an adult's, the trachea is more easily obstructed. Moreover, the pediatric airway has much less cartilaginous support and a larger proportion of soft tissue, rendering it more prone to spasm, collapse or partial collapse. Edema or swelling within the airway can also have much more detrimental effects in a child than in an adult.

Lungs and thorax. Compared to the cone-shaped adult rib case, an infant's rib cage is relatively triangular-shaped. As a result, ventilation occurs through a bellows-like action, as opposed to the piston-like action of the adult diaphragm (see figure 1.6, page 11).

The placement of a tracheostomy tube is much more complex in an infant or child than in an adult for many reasons. Not only is the anatomy much smaller and more compact in infants and children, but the size of the tracheostomy tube cannot change to accommodate the growth of the child's anatomy. For children who require long-term intubation, the tubes must repeatedly be changed to larger sizes to adapt to the child's growing body. At the same time, however, if the child will be fitted with a speaking valve to enable vocalization, then the diameter of the tracheostomy tube must be small enough to allow adequate airflow around the tube and up into the larynx. Finding a balance between adequate respiration and sufficient airflow to allow vocal communication is a frequent dilemma for pediatric speech-language pathologists. The components and placement of alternative airways will be discussed in chapter 3, and chapter 4 is devoted to issues of vocal communication in tracheostomy. First, however, we will review interdisciplinary care concerns for medically complex patients in chapter 2.

Chapter 2

Issues Surrounding Patients with Complex Medical Needs

Patients who do not have a single clear-cut diagnosis with an obvious course of treatment are considered medically complex. These individuals have multiple medical conditions that may compromise their recovery and treatment. Although patients with a tracheostomy tube or ventilator alone have complex needs, their situation can be, and typically is, compounded by other medical issues. This chapter highlights many other areas of a patient's medical status and discusses how those domains may influence treatment goals and the potential for success. A good awareness and understanding of these issues will assist you in providing appropriate services and accurate information to the patient and family. Gaining a complete understanding of a patient's situation requires investigating (through chart reviews, patient histories and interdisciplinary discussions) the nature of the diagnosis, nutritional status, pulmonary or breathing abilities, prior and current levels of function and, for infants or young children, birth history.

Medical Review

A comprehensive perspective of the patient's medical status leads to an efficient and successful plan of treatment. A thorough review of medical records, interviews with the patient or family or both, and ongoing discussions with other professionals involved in the patient's care will guide the direction of treatment. A thorough medical review includes the following components.

Identification of the medical diagnosis. The diagnosis, or identification of the patient's current medical problem or problems, is determined by a physician. Understanding the diagnosis or diagnoses is important when determining a treatment plan.

Date of onset of the medical problem. It is important to know how recently the current medical condition began, as the most progress typically occurs relatively early in the course of recovery; in addition, the more recent the onset, the more immediate the medical issues typically are.

Primary medical history. Knowledge of any secondary incidents that may have occurred at the onset of the current condition or that may have complicated the course of recovery thus far will give you insight into the complexity of the patient's medical status. Common examples include a cerebral vascular accident during or after surgery, acute respiratory failure or instances where the patient has stopped breathing, episodes of high blood pressure, seizures and adverse reactions to medications.

Past medical history. Pre-existing events or conditions may complicate the plan of treatment. For example, diabetes, history of documented strokes, anxiety, use of tobacco products or excessive alcohol use, past head injury, or prior diagnosis of dementia; for children, developmental delays or birth complications may influence treatment decisions.

Prior level of function. Knowing how the patient was functioning prior to the current condition is vital in determining where treatment should begin and what outcome expectations are realistic. For example, it is an unrealistic goal for a patient who was living in an extended-care facility prior to a recent stroke to live independently without outside care after the stroke. A more appropriate goal is to create a plan of care that will enable the patient to return to the facility and to require the same level of assistance as before the stroke. For some patients, it may not even be a realistic goal for them to regain their prior level of functioning.

Child development and birth history. With infants and children, it is important to investigate their developmental history, including any unusual events surrounding the mother's pregnancy, the birth and the hospital stay. One medical complication is intrauterine growth retardation (IUGR), in which a fetus's development slows significantly or stops in utero, possibly indicating a limitation in overall development. Other examples include maternal drug use during pregnancy, maternal fevers or infections during pregnancy, a complicated delivery or emergency cesarean section, and lack of oxygen during fetal development due to the umbilical cord becoming knotted, kinked or wrapped around the fetus's neck.

A commonly used indication of an infant's stability at birth is an Apgar score. An Apgar score is assigned to every infant at one and five minutes after delivery, with some infants also being reassessed ten minutes after delivery. The score is obtained by rating an infant's appearance in terms of skin color, pulse, activity of the arms and legs, and quality of breathing. Each of those five categories are scored zero, one or two points based on specific behaviors or indicators and added together to get the total Apgar score. Table 2.1, page 15, shows the criteria by which points are assigned,

Sign	Score		
	0	1	2
Appearance	Blue or pale	Blue extremities	Pink
Pulse	Absent	Less than 100/min	More than 100/min
Grimace	No response	Grimace	Cough or sneeze
Activity	Limp	Some flexion	Active
Respiration	Absent	Slow/irregular	Good/crying

Table 2.1. Criteria for assigning an Apgar score

with 10 being the highest and most desired score. (This information is also provided as a reproducible page in Appendix A so you can copy it and keep it handy for quick reference.)

The typical infant scores between 8 and 10 at each assessment. It is hoped those who score low (between 0 and 6) initially will receive a more typical score at the five-minute reassessment. Infants who receive low scores and do not recover or recover only minimally after five minutes give physicians cause for concern.

In a medical chart, Apgar scores are usually noted in this manner: ". . . with Apgar 4^1 and 9^5." This indicates a score of 4 at the one-minute assessment and of 9 at the five-minute assessment. The chart will also document any treatment that resulted (for example, ". . . resulting in immediate intubation and ventilator need"). This information will help you formulate an appropriate plan of treatment. For example, a two-year-old child who has been ventilator-dependent since birth is unlikely to succeed with a plan of treatment that requires independent breathing without the ventilator for speech. Such a child would be more successful with a means of vocal communication that is compatible with the ventilator. The information gained from the Apgar score is also important in identifying a child's prior level of function and the strengths on which to base goals. (Note that it is common for communication or swallowing treatment provided by the speech-language pathologist to initiate positive changes in a patient's ventilatory or respiratory status. For example, the speech-language pathologist may recommend trials of a speaking valve while on the ventilator. In accomplishing this goal, the patient may tolerate a decrease in ventilator settings.)

Because a great deal of information must be collected and organized, we have provided a chart review form on page 16, which you may photocopy or use as a model for creating your own form.

Medical History and Chart Review Form

Patient: Patient ID #:	Age: Sex: [ ] F [ ] M	Date of admit:
Diagnosis:		Physician:
Prior level of function/social history:		
Past medical history:		

Birth/Developmental Status

Complications of pregnancy:		
Complications of delivery:		
Gestational age at birth:	Adjusted age:	Apgar scores:
Visual status:	Hearing status:	Alertness:
Physical limitations:		
Cognitive development:		
Developmental milestones:		

Current Pulmonary Status

Trach size/type:	Cuff: [ ] Inflated [ ] Deflated [ ] Cuffless	Fenestrated: [ ] Yes [ ] No
O_2 received via:	Level of O_2 received:	Resting O_2 sats: %
Hrs. of vent need/day:	Mode: Set rate:	Patient-initiated resp. rate:
Tidal volume:	FiO_2: %	Secretions:
[ ] Vent weaning	Hours per day:	Tolerance:

Communication

[ ] Speaking valve type: _____   [ ] Communication device:

[ ] Mouthing words   [ ] Leak speech   [ ] Electrolarynx   [ ] Writing   [ ] Talking Trach

Current Medical Status

Cognitive status:		
Physical limitations:		Activity level:
[ ] Oral diet:	[ ] TPN [ ] Tube fed:	Dental status:
Specific feeding instructions:		
Visual status: [ ] Glasses	Hearing status: [ ] Hearing aids:	

During the chart review and patient/family interview, ask yourself questions that will aid in the formulation of a successful and efficient treatment plan. Here is a list of questions to consider when investigating a patient's history; most will be discussed further in this chapter:

- What is the nature of the diagnosis? Could it be degenerative?

- Why does the individual need a tracheostomy tube or ventilator?

- Has the individual's anatomy changed as a result of his or her current medical status? (For example, placement of a tracheostomy tube alters how a person breathes. Was the tube necessary due to damage to, and thus a change in, the structures around the pharynx or larynx?)

- Will these anatomical changes limit treatment options for communication or swallowing?

- Is the individual's need for respiratory support temporary or long term? If temporary, should treatment be postponed until the patient can support his or her own respiratory needs? What short-term intervention is needed in the interim (e.g., a communication board or yes/no communication system)? If long-term, how can the treatment plan be implemented given the patient's current respiratory status?

- Have there been any attempts to wean the patient from the ventilator (that is, attempts to have the patient breathe without ventilator assistance)? How successful have they been?

- If attempts have been unsuccessful, how does that limit the patient's treatment options? Should treatment be postponed (with appropriate interim interventions) until the patient can breathe independently, or can the treatment plan actually promote weaning?

- Have there been recurrent episodes of aspiration pneumonia or unexplained elevated temperatures? How long has the individual presented with these symptoms?

- Has the individual been evaluated by other medical specialists? If so, what were their recommendations regarding the patient's status and potential?

- For an infant or child, what were the Apgar scores? What do they indicate in terms of the child's ability to sustain adequate respiration?

- What developmental milestones has the infant or child met or failed to meet?

In many cases, not all of your questions can be answered by chart reviews or family interviews. It is important to seek out the expertise of the other professionals involved in the patient's care.

Interdisciplinary Care Team

A variety of professionals are involved in the care of any hospitalized patient, particularly a patient with complex medical needs. Each professional has a unique perspective and area of expertise, and a patient's recovery is most successful when all professionals work together as a team, answering each other's questions, providing insight into treatment plans and offering assistance when needed. At times, questions may arise that require consultation with a professional who is not an active member of the team. In such a case, a consult or referral should be pursued.

Many medical settings have a formalized protocol for interdisciplinary team care, with scheduled team meetings to discuss specific patients. In educational settings, the professionals involved in a student's individualized education plan (IEP) typically meet on a periodic basis. In other treatment settings, meetings may be informal and scheduled only when requested by a member of the team.

The following professionals are frequently members of an interdisciplinary care team.

Primary care physician (PCP). The PCP oversees all aspects of the patient's care, maintaining a comprehensive perspective of the patient's treatment and recovery. The PCP is in charge of recommending specific therapies, changing medications, ordering specific tests and lab work, making referrals to specialists and authorizing specific procedures such as a modified barium swallow study or speaking valve trials. Some PCPs request that a copy of all documentation be sent to them so they can remain informed of the individual's status and progress. A PCP may be a specialist such as an internist (specialist in internal medicine) a pulmonologist or a physiatrist.

Pulmonologist. A pulmonologist is a physician who specializes in the lungs and the function of breathing. He or she determines the parameters of the ventilator settings, the frequency of breathing treatments, the status of the lungs, whether the patient can tolerate trial feedings if aspiration is a risk, and parameters for ventilator or tracheostomy weaning. Some pulmonologists specialize in pediatric care.

Physiatrist or physical medicine and rehabilitation (PM&R) specialist. A physiatrist focuses on a patient's rehabilitation needs, skills and progress. He or she answers questions regarding a patient's potential for rehabilitation, assists in discharge planning, adjusts medications to facilitate higher cognitive functioning, and approves recommendations for treatment such as speaking valve trials, initiation of trial feedings or a modified barium swallow study. If this specialist is not a member of the team at the onset of a patient's treatment, one may be consulted later in the course of recovery.

Neurologist. Neurologists specialize in the brain and its effect on such issues as physical movement, seizure activity, cognition and mental status. They address concerns regarding altered mental status, the potential for the brain to recover its ability to control motor function, whether the patient is competent to make decisions regarding medical intervention and changes in medications for the reduction of anxiety.

Otolaryngologist (Ear, Nose and Throat (ENT) Specialist). An otolaryngologist is an expert regarding complications of the ears, nose and throat. This specialist is a valuable resource when questions arise regarding the patient's laryngeal, audiological or pharyngeal status. For example, an ENT may be consulted to determine whether a patient has vocal cord paralysis or a narrowing of the trachea (also termed tracheal stenosis) that may contraindicate removal of the tracheostomy tube. He or she may order specific audiological tests and may even perform the initial tracheotomy procedure.

Registered nurse. Nurses follow through with a physician's orders for the patient's care. They administer medications, maintain tube feedings, monitor vital signs, and document the growth and development of infants and children. They also assist with daily care and hygiene for patients who are unable to meet these needs independently. Nurses have different levels of responsibility depending on their level of expertise. The registered nurse (RN), the most highly trained nursing professional, is responsible for any invasive medical procedures and for supervision of the nursing staff. The RN typically represents the nursing staff on the interdisciplinary care team. Nursing staff with progressively less expertise are licensed practical nurses (LPNs), patient care technicians (PCTs) and certified nursing assistants (CNAs).

Respiratory therapist (RT). Respiratory therapists take care of the daily management of the patient's pulmonary needs. They administer breathing treatments, clean the tracheostoma site, change the tracheostomy tube, suction the airway when necessary and maintain ventilatory support and weaning parameters as directed by the physician. The RT also assists the speech-language pathologist with swallowing and voice assessments of individuals requiring tracheostomy tubes and those who also need mechanical ventilation.

Occupational therapist (OT). Occupational therapists have a good understanding of the patient's upper extremity skills, ability to perform activities of daily living and visual functioning. For example, they may address the patient's ability to dress and perform daily hygiene routines, facilitate an increase in arm and torso strength, and determine the person's ability to prepare meals safely using kitchen appliances. OTs are frequently a good resource when adaptive equipment must be provided or created, such as determining how a patient could access an alternative means of communication.

Physical therapist (PT). PTs often work in conjunction with OTs. They have a good understanding of a patient's level of endurance and mobility skills, and often work to increase the patient's trunk support. Input from a PT may be especially helpful in adapting seating equipment to facilitate the best postural alignment for the patient when you are working on swallowing and speech goals. Proper postural support facilitates respiratory function and proper alignment of the musculature, laying the foundation for vocal communication and coordination of the swallowing mechanism.

Speech-language pathologist (SLP). SLPs have four areas of focus: cognitive-linguistic skills, facilitation of communication, assessment and treatment of swallowing disorders (dysphagia), and the promotion of developmental skills for infant and pediatric clients. For example, SLPs facilitate an individual's level of orientation, verbal reasoning and problem-solving ability, appropriate use of language, effective communication, safe swallowing, and achievement of developmental speech and language milestones.

Dietitian/Nutritionist. This specialist calculates estimated caloric needs to promote healing and maintain body weight. The dietitian usually recommends the amount and caloric density of alternative nutrition and is helpful in assisting with the transition from alternative nutrition to oral intake.

Social worker/Case manager. This individual assists with discharge planning, arranging the purchase of durable medical equipment and home supplies, and contacting social services to provide needed support after the patient returns home. He or she also acts as a liaison between third-party payers, the facility, and the patient or family. Specially trained social workers or case managers can also assist with meeting the psychosocial and emotional needs of the patient and family.

Understanding the Nature of the Diagnosis

Many diseases can interfere with the ability to breathe either temporarily or permanently. The nature of these conditions may be traumatic or acute (a sudden onset of symptoms), pulmonary (respiratory in nature), neuromuscular (affecting muscle control dictated by the brain), or congenital (present at birth). A strong understanding of the nature of the diagnosis ensures an accurate appraisal of the patient and development of an appropriate treatment plan.

When a patient has undergone a traumatic event, such as a motor vehicle accident, gunshot wound or significant burn injury, the diagnosis is considered traumatic or acute. This means that the person had a sudden change in life resulting in the present condition. An example of a traumatic condition that may interfere with respiration is acute traumatic brain injury due to a car accident in which the brain suffered such trauma as to cause the cessation of breathing. In this case, respiratory failure, or apnea, is a direct result of the brain injury. A gunshot wound to the chest or neck may alter a patient's anatomy, rendering him or her unable to breathe effectively or efficiently. Similarly, smoke inhalation during a fire may irritate the lungs and decrease respiratory efficiency, creating the temporary need for an alternative means of respiration, such as a ventilator. In all these examples, one can assume (unless otherwise noted in the medical history) that the patient's anatomy was typical prior to the traumatic event. Such information is important when discussing options for treatment of communication and swallowing, since an atypical anatomical foundation most likely will limit the options for treatment. Such a dilemma may be present in cases of congenital diagnoses.

In a congenital diagnosis, the medical complications were diagnosed either in utero or at birth and may have interfered with the typical development of the individual's brain, bones, muscles or organs. Many congenital syndromes involve anatomical changes to the respiratory and airway systems. Some are severe enough to alter the bone structure of the face, mouth, hard palate and trachea, thus affecting the individual's ability to speak effectively or swallow safely. When attempting to create a plan of treatment for an individual with a congenital diagnosis, it is usually helpful to review diagnostic images and procedure reports such as x-rays, brain scans, videofluoroscopies and laryngoscopies (in which a small camera is passed into the larynx to observe the function of the vocal cords and the patency, or openness, of the trachea).

When the condition involves a disease process, as is typical with pulmonary and neuromuscular diagnoses, the creation of a direct plan of care is complicated. This is especially true when the disease is progressive and an overall decline in the patient's function is inevitable. In such cases, the plan of treatment is ever-changing and is based on the patient's current level of function at a particular time, changing repeatedly as the patient's abilities become more and more limited. A specific example is amyotrophic lateral sclerosis (ALS, or Lou Gehrig's disease). As the disease progresses over time, the ability to breathe independently declines until the body is unable to sustain adequate ventilation on its own. The need for artificial ventilation may lead to new concerns regarding communication and the safety of swallowing that were not present initially. A solid understanding of the diagnosis and course of any progressive disease is imperative in determining short- and long-term goals and educating the patient and family on the overall prognosis and plan of treatment.

Nutritional Status

It is important to know how a patient is receiving his or her nutrition. There are three ways of maintaining nutrition: orally (eating food by mouth), intravenously (bypassing the entire gastric system with liquid nutrition though the veins), or by different forms of tube feeding (placing liquid nutrition into the stomach and thus bypassing the swallowing mechanism). Sometimes the type of diagnosis will suggest the patient's future nutritional status. For example, a patient with a traumatic diagnosis may receive tube feedings initially but with therapy probably will return to oral feedings as recovery progresses, whereas a patient with a chronic disease process may have a much poorer prognosis. Helping a patient return to oral feedings is usually the goal of treatment. Some patients may need to depend on other forms of nutrition and hydration until that goal can be realized, however, and others may be dependent permanently on an alternative or supplemental form of nutrition and hydration, if the safety and efficiency of their swallowing function is a concern.

Intravenous nutrition, also called TPN for total parenteral nutrition, is most often used when the digestive tract must be bypassed for some reason; for example, during surgery or because the patient cannot metabolize nutrition through the gastric system. The need for this type of nutrition may be temporary or long term. Because swallowing ability is irrelevant if the patient cannot digest the swallowed food properly, it is important to determine the overall prognosis for gastric function (which usually requires a discussion with a gastroenterologist, or GI specialist). Because swallowing trials require introducing food into the gastric system, it is imperative that the system be functioning. If the GI specialist states that no means of nutrition other than TPN is permissible, swallowing function cannot be assessed. If the system is being bypassed only temporarily, the swallowing evaluation is postponed until the GI specialist gives the approval to proceed.

When tube feeding is used, several placements are possible, depending on the length of time alternative nutrition will be needed (see figure 2.1). Typically, if the need is short term, a tube is temporarily placed either down the nose or through the mouth, into the esophagus and into the gastric system. These types of tubes are either a nasogastric tube (NG tube or NGT) or a duotube (also referred to as a Dobhoff Tube or DHT). They differ in the following ways: A duotube is smaller in diameter and more flexible than the NGT, and it has a weighted tip that helps to place it in the duodenum (the upper part of the small intestine) and maintain its position there. The NGT, which terminates in the stomach, is not weighted and has greater potential for movement. The placement of a duotube must be checked radiographically before it can be used for nutrition, which is unnecessary for an NG tube. The PCP will order a specific procedure called a KUB (for "kidney, ureter and bladder," which is similar to an x-ray of the abdomen) to make sure that the weighted tip is located in the duodenum. In contrast, the positioning of an NG tube can be checked by a nurse at bedside. While placing a stethoscope over the stomach, the nurse injects a small amount of air into the tube and listens for the resulting puff in the stomach to verify that it is placed correctly. Although the duotube is more easily inserted and is more comfortable for the patient, its primary

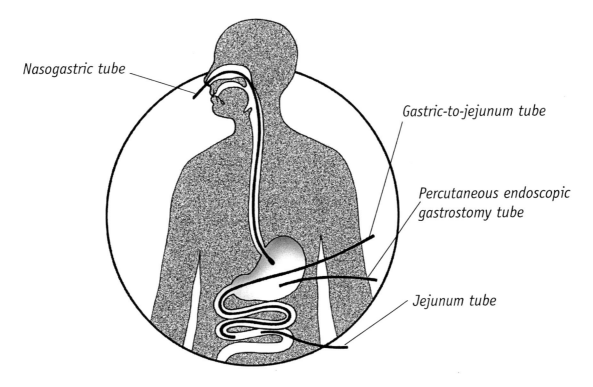

Nasogastric tube

Gastric-to-jejunum tube

Percutaneous endoscopic gastrostomy tube

Jejunum tube

Figure 2.1. Gastrointestinal system, showing placements of nasogastric tube, gastric-to-jejunum (G-J) tube, percutaneous endoscopic gastrostomy tube (PEG), jejunum tube (J)

disadvantage is the cost of the KUB to check placement every time it must be replaced.

A long-term means of alternative nutrition is a feeding tube surgically placed into the stomach or intestine through the abdominal wall. There are several types of such tubes; a percutaneous endoscopic gastrostomy tube (PEG or G tube) is inserted directly into the stomach. A tube placed directly into the intestines is inserted into the jejunum (the part of the intestine just past the duodenum) and is referred to as a jejunum tube (J tube). Another option is a G-J tube (for gastric to jejunum tube), in which the tube initially is inserted into the stomach and is then fed into the jejunum.

There may be several reasons why it is necessary to place a feeding tube in the intestines rather than the stomach, as determined by the GI specialist. Common reasons include a high incidence of gastroesophageal reflux disease (GERD), continuing emesis (vomiting), or chronic aspiration of the reflux or emesis. Placing the feeding tube into the intestinal tract rather than the stomach increases the distance from the esophagus, decreasing the likelihood that the feeding will travel that far.

Regardless of the means by which the patient receives nutrition, another significant issue to consider is whether the patient has a solid nutritional foundation to support the treatment plan. A good nutritional foundation promotes healing and recovery. An individual who has been losing weight since admission or is not receiving sufficient nutrition may not be a candidate to begin treatment until a good nutritional foundation can be maintained. A discussion with the dietitian can reveal whether the patient is receiving adequate nutrition to promote recovery.

Respiratory Status

It is important to determine the underlying stability of the respiratory system. Humans need a specific amount of oxygen to maintain basic body functions. Regular environmental air (sometimes referred to as room air) contains an average of 21 percent oxygen. Individuals who are not medically compromised are able to maintain adequate oxygenation of their blood (typically 92 to 98 percent oxygenation) by breathing room air.

Some individuals are unable to maintain that level without supplemental oxygen. It is possible to breathe up to 100 percent (pure) oxygen if a physician determines this is necessary to support bodily functions. However, the higher the level of supplemental oxygen needed, the less stable and efficient the patient's pulmonary status. As a general rule of thumb, any patient who is dependent on more than 40 percent oxygen is considered too heavily dependent or compromised to successfully tolerate changes in the plan of care. It is usually necessary to wait until the patient can be weaned to a lower level of supplemental oxygen before initiating treatment. To attempt treatment too early may stress the patient's endurance to the limit, resulting in failure. A team consultation (particularly with the pulmonologist and respiratory therapist) will determine the person's status, weaning potential, and treatment possibilities.

Monitoring the Individual with Complex Medical Needs

Monitoring the patient's status before, during and after treatment will alert you to the patient's readiness for treatment, ability to tolerate treatment, and success or limitations in response to the treatment. At times, monitoring may reveal specific times when the patient is performing at his or her best; if so, it may be beneficial to reschedule treatments to coincide with those times. The following techniques are options for monitoring a patient's respiratory status; some require special equipment that may not be available during all treatment sessions (see Appendix B for a vendor list). Normal values for most of these measures are also provided as reproducible pages in Appendix A (see pages 135-136), which you may copy and keep handy for quick reference.

Facial Coloring and Skin Temperature

Equipment needed: none

Procedure: Observe the patient's face

Typical: Skin color is healthy, with pinkish cheeks and lips; skin should be cool to warm to the touch.

Atypical: Skin is pale or dusky-colored, with pale or gray lips; patient sweats visibly; skin is cool or clammy to the touch.

Intervention: Alert the caregiver or nurse taking care of the individual; reschedule treatment for a later time or another day; assist other team members with any directed ventilation techniques or temperature-regulation procedures as needed.

Breathing and Respiratory Rate

Equipment needed: Pulse oximeter

Procedure: Place the pulse oximeter on one finger or, for an infant, around the width of the foot (see figure 2.2, page 26); this is a non-invasive procedure that speech-language pathologists can use. If no equipment is available, simply count the number of breaths per minute. Also observe the nature of the patient's breathing.

Typical: Adults have an average resting breath rate of twelve to twenty breaths per minute (bpm); the average for children ranges from thirty to forty bpm; and infants range from sixty to eighty bpm. Breathing should be rhythmical, with bilateral chest expansion; the patient should be able to breathe easily through both the mouth and nose.

Atypical: Breaths per minute are significantly above or below the norm; breathing is shallow and rapid; patient uses atypical breathing patterns:

- *Neck breathing:* the accessory muscles of the neck and shoulders contract visibly during inhalation.

- *Belly breathing*: The stomach distends noticeably with each breath.

- *Paradoxical breathing*: The chest rises as the stomach falls and vice versa.

- *Guppy breathing*: The mouth is wide open and the individual appears to be gasping for air.

- *Effortful breathing*: Every breath appears to be a challenge.

- *Minimal breathing*: Little breath flow can be felt from either the mouth or nose.

Intervention: Alert the nurse or caregiver. Attempt to calm the patient if the respiratory rate is high or to arouse the patient if respiratory rate is low. If atypical breathing patterns are present, attempt to redirect the patient to a more typical breathing technique. If the patient is using a speaking valve, remove the valve. Assist other profes-

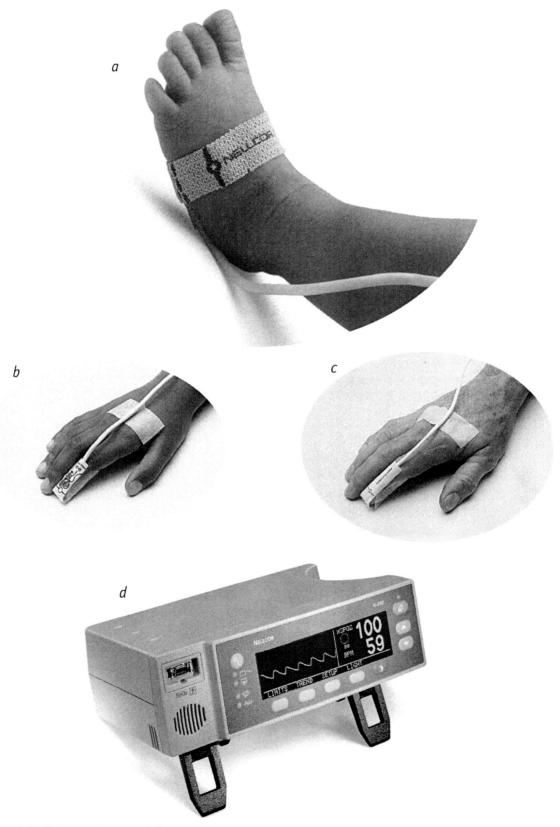

Figure 2.2. Pulse oximetry: (a) neonate sensor; (b) pediatric sensor; (c) adult sensor; and (d) monitor. (Reprinted by permission of Nellcor Puritan Bennett, Inc., Pleasanton, CA.)

sionals with any directed ventilation procedures as needed.

Pulse Rate

Equipment needed: pulse oximeter (optional)

Procedure: Place the pulse oximeter on one finger or, for an infant, around the foot (see figure 2.2). If no equipment is available, count the radial pulse manually by placing two fingers over the patient's radial (wrist) pulse points and counting the pulse rate for one minute (or count for thirty seconds and multiply by two). Although there are quicker ways to obtain a pulse rate, this method will give more accurate insight into the patient's cardiac activity, as many medically complex patients have weak or sporadic pulses.

Typical: Neonates average 120 to 160 heartbeats per minute; children range from 80 to 140; young adults range from 75 to 100 and adults range from 60 to 100 heartbeats per minute.

Atypical: Pulse rates are significantly higher or lower than the average range for your patient's age.

Intervention: Alert the caregiver or nurse. Attempt to calm the patient if the heart rate is high. If the patient is using a speaking valve, remove the valve.

Oxygen Saturation Level

Equipment needed: pulse oximeter or lab results from an immediate arterial blood gas (ABG) draw ordered by a physician

Procedure: Place the pulse oximeter on one index finger (see figure 2.2). In an ABG draw, a nurse or respiratory therapist draws blood from a peripheral artery (usually in the wrist) and sends it immediately to the lab for analysis of oxygen and carbon dioxide, acidity and tension levels, all of which are measures of blood oxygenation.

Typical: The ideal range for all ages is 92 to 100 percent oxygen saturation as recorded on the pulse oximeter. The range of normal results of an ABG are as follows:

Oxygen saturation (SaO_2):	97–98%
Peripheral arterial oxygenation (PaO_2):	80–100 mm Hg
Peripheral arterial carbon dioxide ($PaCO_2$):	35–45 mm Hg
Blood acidity (pH):	7.35–7.45

Atypical: Saturation levels lower than 88 percent or that continue to drop rather than stabilizing or rising; the following atypical ABG results may indicate respiratory distress:

- *Acidosis*: ABG results showing pH < 7.35, $PaCO_2$ > 45 mm Hg and PaO_2 < 80 mm Hg may indicate excessive carbon dioxide retention in the blood (acidosis). Mechanical ventilation may be required to clear out the carbon dioxide before it can reach a poisonous level that would affect tissue, organ and brain functions. Physical symptoms may include quick bounding pulse, rapid and shallow respiration, lethargy, confusion, dizziness or headache. Also monitor the patient's level of alertness, as another symptom of carbon dioxide retention is decreased alertness and slowing of cognitive functions. (If this behavior occurs while the pulse oximeter or ABG shows oxygenation levels to be within normal range, there is cause for concern.)

- *Alkalosis*: ABG results showing $pH > 7.45$, $PaCO_2 < 35$ mm Hg and $PaO_2 < 60$ mm Hg may indicate a lack of oxygen in the blood (alkalosis), meaning that insufficient oxygen is reaching the tissues, organs and brain to meet metabolic needs. Again, mechanical ventilation may be indicated to regain adequate oxygenation. Physical symptoms may include headache, irritability, dizziness, slowed pulse and tingling of the extremities.

Intervention: Alert the nurse, respiratory therapist or caregiver to any behavioral signs. If the patient is using a speaking valve, remove the valve. Suction the airway if necessary and reschedule treatment when respiratory status is stabilized. Assist other team members with directed ventilation techniques as needed.

In addition to monitoring the patient's condition before, during and after treatment, it is important to note how long it takes the patient to "recover" from the treatment sessions. The patient's medical status takes priority over the treatment schedule: treatment may be unsuccessful or even counterproductive if it takes the patient a considerable amount of time, energy and cognitive reorganization to recover from the effort of participating in therapy.

When in doubt about a patient's status, it is always better to ask for assistance than to ignore atypical signs you observe. If you are working in a patient's home, there may be no medical professionals on-site. Placing a call to the home health agency to consult with a nurse or respiratory therapist may be warranted. Sometimes a phone call to the patient's physician regarding treatment results and concerns is appropriate and appreciated. Finally, all speech-language pathologists should remain current in cardiopulmonary resuscitation (CPR) and artificial resuscitation skills, especially those working with medically complex patients.

Conclusion

Although the task of piecing together a complex medical history may seem time consuming, even daunting perhaps, doing so offers better insight into the patient's current status, immediate medical needs and treatment potential. It is imperative to have a thorough understanding of the nature of the patient's diagnosis; to monitor the individual before, during and after treatment sessions; and to develop a relationship with the other team members. *The patient's status always takes priority in the setting of goals and scheduling of treatment sessions.* If the patient has more urgent issues than swallowing or speaking (such as limited respiratory support or a poor nutritional foundation), it is in the patient's best interest to wait until those issues are resolved, or at least stabilized, before beginning treatment. Maintaining a global perspective of each patient will help you develop the most successful treatment plan.

Chapter 3
Alternative Airways

Although a speech-language pathologist is accustomed to assisting adults and children with swallowing and communication deficits, the introduction of an endotracheal or tracheostomy tube presents a new set of issues and concerns. Understanding the components of various tubes and the different implications of orally and nasally placed endotracheal tubes versus tracheotomy-placed tubes will allow a clinician to provide the best possible service to the patient. In this chapter we will discuss the reasons individuals may require oral or nasal intubation or tracheotomy, and the procedures for placement of these tubes.

Types of Intubation

The placement of a tube in a hollow organ or body passage is referred to as intubation. Airway intubation is necessary for patients who require assistance with breathing or with maintaining adequate oxygenation. It is necessary to ensure a patent (open) airway for the respiratory system in order to sustain life. Frequently intubation is done in an emergency situation, with the primary concern being to place the tube as quickly as possible in order to assist ventilation.

There are three types of intubation: two short-term (typically fourteen to twenty-one days) and one long-term. For short-term respiratory management, an endotracheal (ET) tube can be placed either through the oral cavity (called oral intubation) or the nasal cavity (called nasal intubation) to facilitate airway management and secretion removal (see figure 3.1, page 32). Should the individual require long-term airway management, a tracheostomy tube can be placed directly into the trachea in an operation called a tracheotomy.

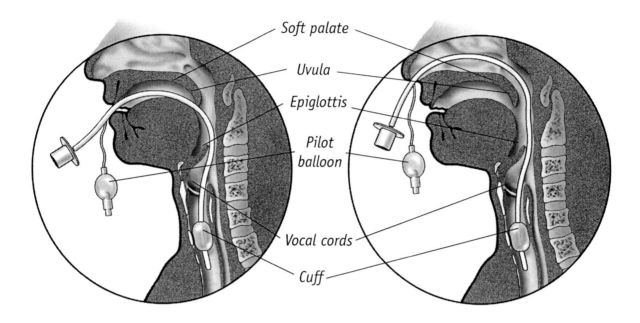

Soft palate
Uvula
Epiglottis
Pilot balloon
Vocal cords
Cuff

Figure 3.1. Lateral view of oral and nasal endotracheal intubation.

Placement of an oral ET tube is performed by trained medical personnel such as physicians or respiratory therapists. The individual is placed in a supine position with the head hyperextended in an effort to straighten the airway as much as possible. The hyperextension must be done with extreme caution. If the individual has suffered a cervical spinal injury, this position could further the injury, perhaps causing permanent paralysis. While using a laryngoscope to visualize the true vocal cords, the physician slides the ET tube over the base of the tongue, through the glottis between the vocal cords and into the trachea. Placement of an ET tube nasally is performed in essentially the same manner except that the ET tube is passed through the nares and a rigid or flexible bronchoscope is used to visualize the vocal cords.

Once either type of ET tube is in place, a soft plastic ring on the tube, called a cuff, is inflated, helping to anchor the tube in place and to create a seal between the lungs and the upper airway. Without this seal, oxygen introduced through the tube would escape into the oral cavity and would be of little benefit to the patient. If the breathing difficulty was caused by obstruction of the airway, the patient may begin breathing independently. If not, the ET tube can be immediately connected to a manual resuscitation bag for temporary breathing assistance (see figure 3.2), or to a ventilator for longer-term needs. A respiratory therapist (RT) will set up and monitor the ventilator according to the physician's orders and specifications.

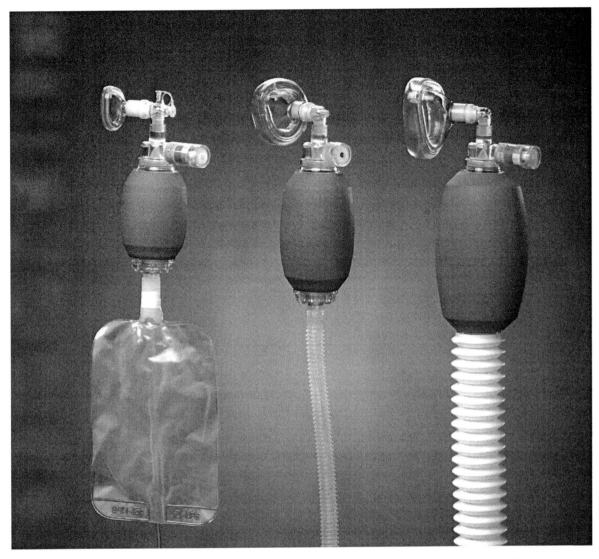

Figure 3.2. Manual resuscitation bag. (Reprinted by permission of Nellcor Puritan Bennett, Inc., Pleasanton, CA.)

Several complications may result from oral or nasal ET tube placement. These include trauma to the oral, nasal, laryngeal or pharyngeal structures, including necrosis (tissue death), granulation tissue (damaged tissue attempting to heal), granulomas (swollen masses of granulation tissue) or laryngeal webbing (growth of tissue in the larynx that partially occludes the glottis). Other possible complications are glottal incompetence (inability to adduct the vocal cords), hypoxemia (insufficient oxygenation of the blood), cardiac complications, lung collapse or damage to the esophagus.

Individuals who are orally or nasally intubated cannot swallow safely or communicate vocally. Because the ET tube blocks the oral or nasal cavity and maintains an open glottis, speaking is impossible and swallowing is contraindicated; it is important that the person remains strictly NPO (nothing by mouth) until the tube is removed. The greatest service you can offer from a treatment perspective is to provide an interim means of communication, if the patient is sufficiently awake and alert to communicate. Mitsuda and colleagues (1992) relate several case studies of patients who suffered needless pain and anxiety because of their inability to communicate. For example, one woman was intubated for nine days with her eyes swollen shut. In response to her evident pain, the physicians repeatedly increased her morphine doses. After the tube was removed, she was finally able to communicate that she had mascara in her eyes! There are several resources for augmentative communication. A temporary communication system could be as simple as a hand-squeezing or eye-blink system for yes/no responses or topic selection. More versatile is a pointing or eye-gaze board with letters or words, or even an electronic augmentative communication system. (Alternative communication is covered in more detail in chapter 4.)

Tracheotomy Procedure

If an individual is going to require relatively long-term intubation, or if there is a blockage in the oral cavity, pharynx or larynx, a tracheostomy tube will most likely be placed. A fundamental difference between a tracheostomy tube and an ET tube is that of placement. Whereas the ET tube is inserted between the vocal cords, the tracheostomy tube is inserted into the trachea below the level of the vocal cords. Thus, barring other medical issues, a person with a tracheostomy tube may be able to swallow normally. The person also may be able to adduct the vocal cords for protection of the airway and to speak if airflow is directed upward through the larynx.

There are two methods of placing a tracheostomy tube, both of which under typical circumstances require trained medical personnel. The procedure used is strictly up to the physician's personal preference and training. The most common and traditional method is a surgical procedure called a tracheotomy, in which a lateral incision is made at the level of either the second and third or third and fourth tracheal rings, just below the level of the vocal cords. The tracheostomy tube is then inserted (see figure 3.3) and secured around the person's neck with fabric or hook-and-loop fastener (such as Velcro®) ties. Sutures may be necessary to close the tracheostoma (opening) around the tracheostomy tube.

The second method of tracheostomy tube placement is percutaneous placement, a relatively new procedure that is gaining popularity in the medical field. In the percutaneous procedure, a small incision is made in the trachea, then a series of dilators are used to gradually increase the size of the tracheostoma (referred to as serial dilation). When the tracheostoma has been dilated to the specified size, a specialized

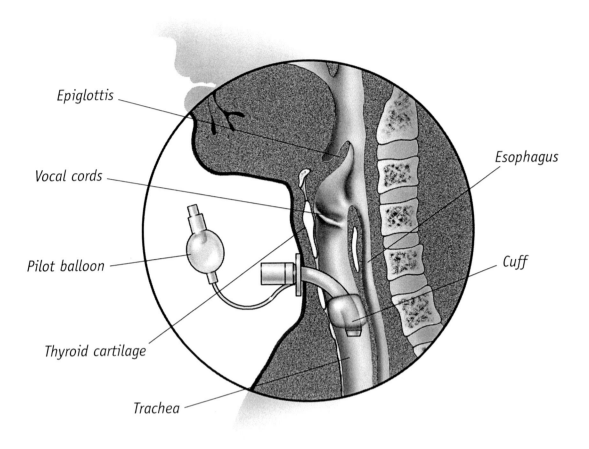

Figure 3.3. Lateral view of tracheostomy tube, with cuff inflated.

tracheostomy tube is inserted. This specialized percutaneous tube is more flexible than other brands and fits more precisely within the tracheostoma (see figure 3.4), but it is placed in the manner described previously. The percutaneous procedure has other advantages as well: it can be done at bedside and does not require a surgical suite; the procedure lasts only twenty to thirty minutes; the tracheostoma size is more precise, thus reducing or eliminating the need for sutures; and there tends to be less bleeding.

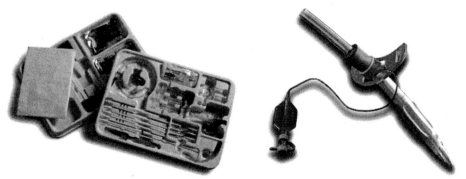

Figure 3.4. Portex percutaneous tracheotomy kit and percutaneous tracheostomy tube. (Courtesy of Portex, Inc.)

Components of a Tracheostomy Tube

There are many different manufacturers of tracheostomy tubes. Each brand of tube has some unique characteristics and qualities. Physicians may also choose particular brands based on their individual preferences as well. Generally, however, all tubes have the same basic parts:

■ Outer Cannula

The outer cannula is the main part of the tracheostomy tube (see figure 3.5). The shaft of the outer cannula is what maintains the patency (openness) of the tracheostoma and provides access to the respiratory system. The outer cannula may be fenestrated or unfenestrated (with or without holes). The purpose of these openings on the top side of the shaft is to allow increased airflow into the pharynx.

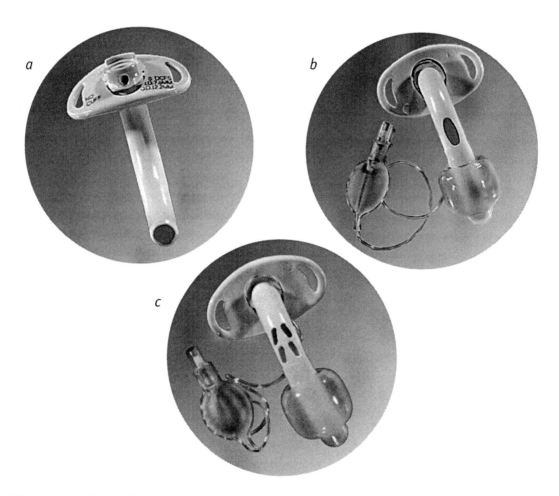

Figure 3.5. (a) Unfenestrated outer cannula; (b) outer cannula with a single fenestration; and (c) outer cannula with multiple fenestrations. (Reprinted by permission of Nellcor Puritan Bennett, Inc., Pleasanton, CA.)

Inner Cannula

The inner cannula is a tube that matches the shape of the outer cannula and is sized to fit inside it. The inner cannula facilitates cleaning of the tracheostomy tube. Mucus tends to collect inside the inner cannula, and it can be easily removed for cleaning or can be discarded and replaced with a fresh one. The inner cannula also may be fenestrated or unfenestrated to match the specification of the outer cannula (see figure 3.6). Note that not all tracheostomy tubes have inner cannulas. (This is particularly true of neonatal and pediatric tracheostomy tubes, which are often too small in diameter to accommodate an inner cannula).

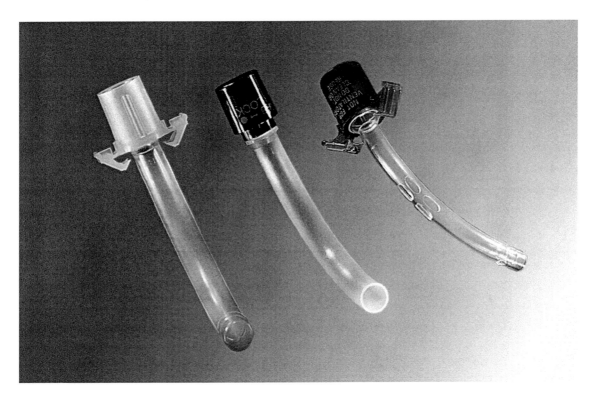

Figure 3.6. Fenestrated and unfenestrated inner cannulas. (Reprinted by permission of Nellcor Puritan Bennett, Inc., Pleasanton, CA.)

Flange and Neck Strap

The flange, or neck plate, is a flat plate that lies against the patient's neck, with slots for insertion of a neck strap. Its primary function is to anchor the outer end of the tracheostomy tube so it cannot fall into the trachea. Information about the tracheostomy tube—manufacturer, type and size—can usually be found on the flange.

Used to secure the tracheostomy tube in place, the neck strap is threaded through the slots on the flange or neck plate. The strap is fastened around the patient's neck with a strip of hook-and-loop fastener (such as Velcro®) or cloth tape.

■ Hub

The hub is the protruding end of the inner cannula and serves as a point of connection between the tracheostomy tube and a ventilator or speaking valve (see figure 3.7). The standard hub is 15 mm in diameter and has a lock to secure the inner cannula to the outer cannula. The disposable inner cannula has a pinch-type lock, whereas the non-disposable inner cannula has a twisting-type lock.

Be aware that the metal tracheostomy tube has what is termed a low-profile hub, which is not the standard 15 mm size and prevents connection to most speaking valves and all ventilators. Some manufacturers will produce, through special order, an inner cannula with a 15 mm hub that will accommodate standard speaking valves (see chapter 4 for further discussion).

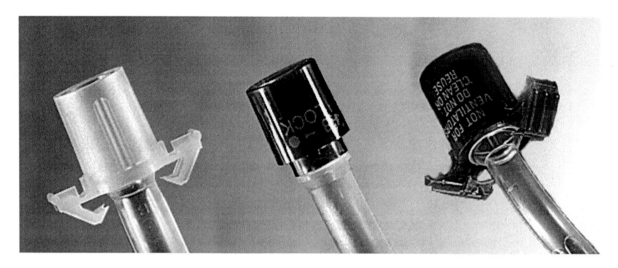

Figure 3.7. Standard 15 mm tracheostomy hub. (Reprinted by permission of Nellcor Puritan Bennett, Inc., Pleasanton, CA.)

■ Cuff and Pilot Balloon

The cuff is an inner-tube-like plastic ring present on some types of tracheostomy tubes (see figure 3.8). This air-filled or foam-filled ring serves two functions: (a) to seal the airway, preventing ventilated air from escaping the lungs, and (b) to act as protection for the airway by making it more difficult for any aspirated material to enter into the lungs (even a properly inflated cuff does not offer complete protection, however, as will be discussed in chapter 5). The pilot balloon is a plastic sac connected via an inflation line (narrow tubing) to the cuff. The pilot balloon allows medical personnel to determine whether the cuff is inflated or deflated. (If the pilot balloon is inflated, so is the cuff, and vice versa.) The cuff is inflated or deflated using a syringe. A spring-loaded valve on the end of the pilot balloon, called a Luer valve, prevents air

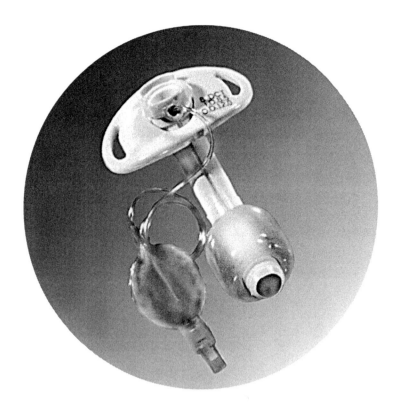

Figure 3.8. Cuff and pilot balloon, shown inflated. (Reprinted by permission of Nellcor Puritan Bennett, Inc., Pleasanton, CA.)

from escaping out of the pilot balloon, which would cause the cuff to deflate. Knowing whether the cuff is inflated or deflated is especially important when considering vocal communication and swallowing therapies for reasons that will be discussed in detail in chapters 4 and 5. Patients may also find the mass of a partially deflated or overinflated cuff uncomfortable. Some tracheostomy tubes are cuffless, in which case they lack both the cuff and pilot balloon.

In most settings, it is the respiratory therapist who inflates and deflates the cuff of a tracheostomy tube and maintains the specified pressure using a manometer. Correct inflation of the cuff is extremely important as an underinflated or overinflated cuff can cause significant complications. An underinflated cuff will allow air to escape upward through the larynx as well as allowing aspirated material to enter the lungs (see figure 3.9, page 40). An overinflated cuff tends to push the posterior wall of the trachea into the esophageal wall, possibly causing fistulas, necrosis, and perhaps increased difficulty with swallowing (see figure 3.10, page 40).

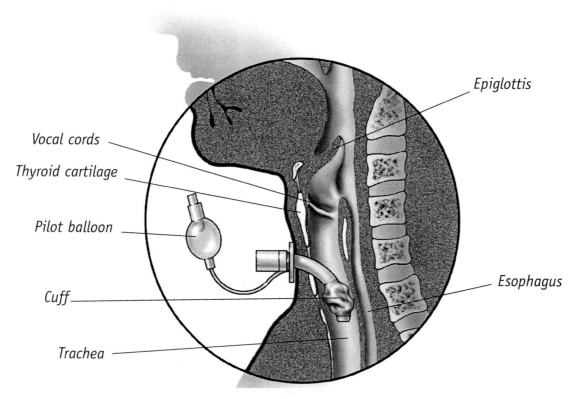

Epiglottis

Vocal cords

Thyroid cartilage

Pilot balloon

Esophagus

Cuff

Trachea

Figure 3.9. Underinflated cuff.

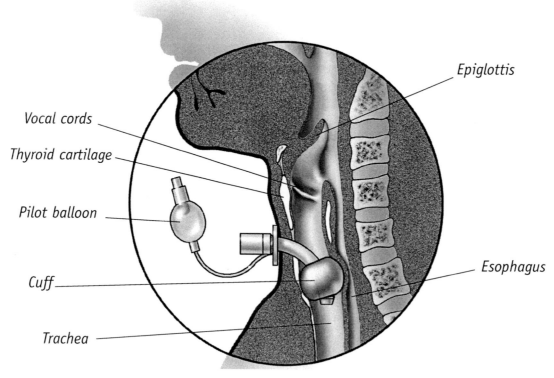

Epiglottis

Vocal cords

Thyroid cartilage

Pilot balloon

Esophagus

Cuff

Trachea

Figure 3.10. Overinflated cuff.

The Bivona Fome-Cuf® brand tracheostomy tubes deserve special mention because they have certain unique features with regard to the cuff and pilot balloon. As the name implies, the cuff is filled with foam and requires the specially provided syringe and attachment for inflation and deflation (see figure 3.11). A characteristic of this foam-filled cuff is that it inflates independently over time (called pressure inflation). In addition, the pilot balloon does not inflate and deflate like other brands, so it is impossible to determine the status of the cuff from looking at the pilot balloon. The pressure-inflation characteristic is optimal for certain patients requiring low cuff pressure to be maintained against the tracheal wall, and it is preferred by some physicians. Its use is contraindicated, however, when the patient is using a speaking valve. (See chapter 4 for further discussion.)

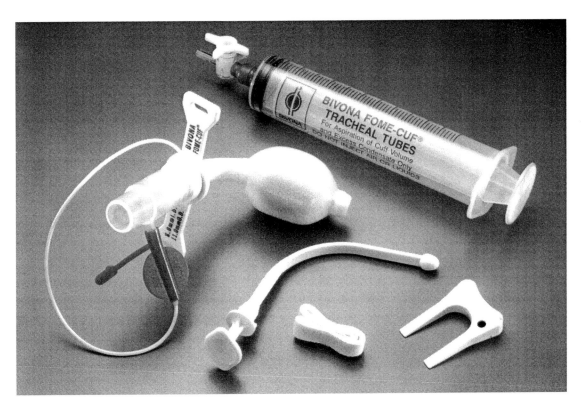

Figure 3.11. Bivona Fome-Cuf® tracheostomy tube. (Courtesy of Bivona Medical Technologies)

▪ Obturator

The obturator is used as a guide during placement of the tracheostomy tube into the airway. It must be removed immediately after placement to allow air to flow through the tube (see figure 3.12, page 42). This part is saved, sterilized and used again should the tracheostomy tube accidentally be removed and need to be replaced.

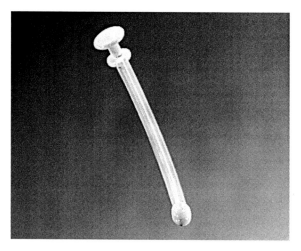

Figure 3.12. Obturator. (Reprinted by permission of Nellcor Puritan Bennett, Inc., Pleasanton, CA.)

Button

The component known variously as a button, plug, cork, or cap completely occludes the end of the tracheostomy tube, allowing the patient to bypass the tube and breathe through the mouth and nose (figure 3.13). Trials with a button or cap constitute one of the steps toward removal of a tracheostomy tube. The button can be removed should the individual require suctioning or should access to the airway become necessary.

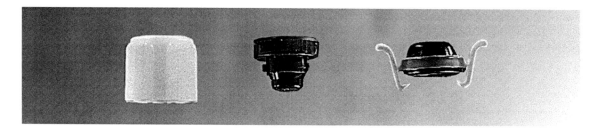

Figure 3.13. Button, plug, cork or cap. (Reprinted by permission of Nellcor Puritan Bennett, Inc., Pleasanton, CA.)

Humidification System

In order to keep the mucosal lining of the trachea and lungs moist, individuals with tracheostomy tubes may need to be connected to a humidification system. There are two basic means of providing artificial humidification. Patients who have an open tracheostomy tube may utilize a tracheostomy collar, a masklike device that is strapped around the individual's neck and loosely covers the tracheostomy tube (see figure 3.14). This device more precisely directs the humidified air toward the tracheostomy tube. Patients who are relatively stable medically may be candidates for a heat–moisture-exchange device (HME), commonly called an artificial nose. This small plastic device attaches to the hub of the tracheostomy tube to filter the air and retain moisture in the respiratory system (see figure 3.15). The advantage of the artificial nose is that the person does not require additional humidification from an outside source, allowing more independence and mobility.

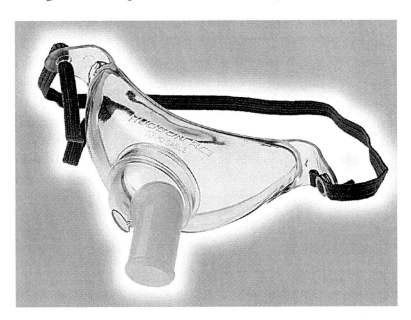

Figure 3.14. Tracheostomy collar or mask. (Courtesy of Medline Industries, Inc.)

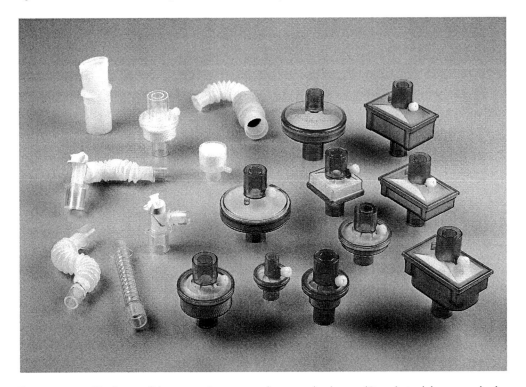

Figure 3.15. Variety of heat-moisture exchange devices. (Reprinted by permission of Nellcor Puritan Bennett, Inc., Pleasanton, CA.)

Components of an Endotracheal Tube

Just as with tracheostomy tubes, there are several different types of ET tubes. The basic ET tube consists of a silicone or polyvinyl chloride (PVC) tube, beveled tip, cuff, pilot balloon, and hub (see figure 3.16). These parts function in a similar manner as their counterparts in a tracheostomy tube. The single most obvious difference between an ET tube and a tracheostomy tube is length, with the ET tube being significantly longer. As discussed earlier in this chapter, the placement is also different, being through the mouth or nose rather than through the trachea.

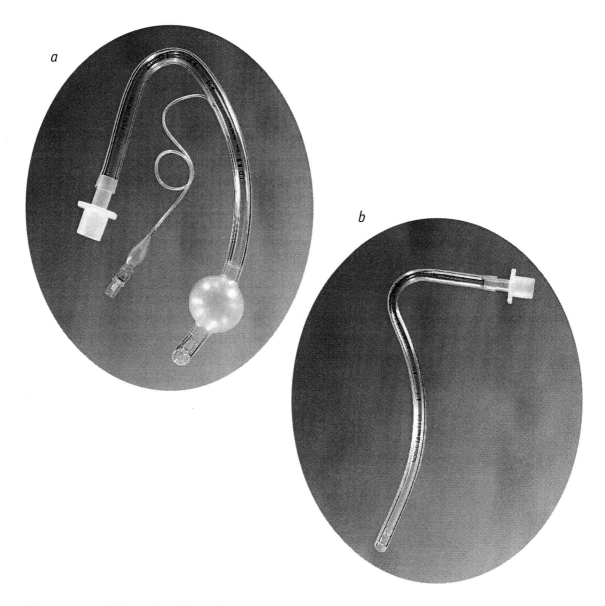

Figure 3.16. (a) Oral endotracheal tube; and (b) cuffless, nasal endotracheal tube. (Reprinted by permission of Nellcor Puritan Bennett, Inc., Pleasanton, CA.)

Alternative Airways

Types of Tracheostomy Tubes

There are different types of tracheostomy tubes, which can be differentiated by the characteristics of their components.

Single Versus Double Cannula

A tracheostomy tube may have only an outer (single) cannula or may have both outer and inner cannulas (double cannula). Double-cannula tracheostomy tubes are used most frequently, but single-cannula tracheostomy tubes are used in special circumstances, usually with infants or children. The use of a double cannula enables easier maintenance of the airway and can allow the patient to play an active role in tracheostomy management. Training the individual to remove his or her inner cannula for cleaning or replacement promotes independence and active participation in long-term medical care (See chapter 7).

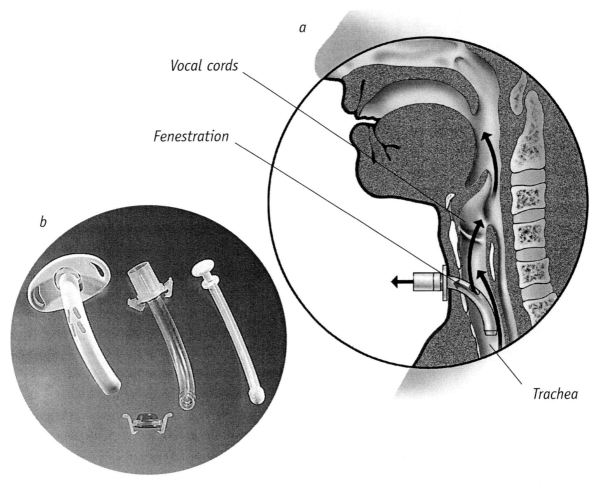

Figure 3.17. A cuffless fenestrated tracheostomy tube: (a) in situ showing placement and airflow; and (b) components. (Reprinted by permission of Nellcor Puritan Bennett, Inc., Pleasanton, CA.)

■ Cuffed Versus Cuffless

As mentioned previously, a tracheostomy tube may or may not have a cuff that seals the trachea (see figures 3.17–3.20, pages 45-47, for examples of both types). A cuff provides protection for the airway and is necessary to prevent air escape if the patient is on a ventilator. A cuffless tracheostomy tube permits upward airflow around the outside of the tube and is used when the potential for aspiration or the need for mechanical ventilation is minimal. Whether the tracheostomy tube is cuffed or cuffless will be printed on the flange. The pilot balloon is another way to identify a cuffed tracheostomy tube because, as you will recall, a cuffless tube has no pilot balloon.

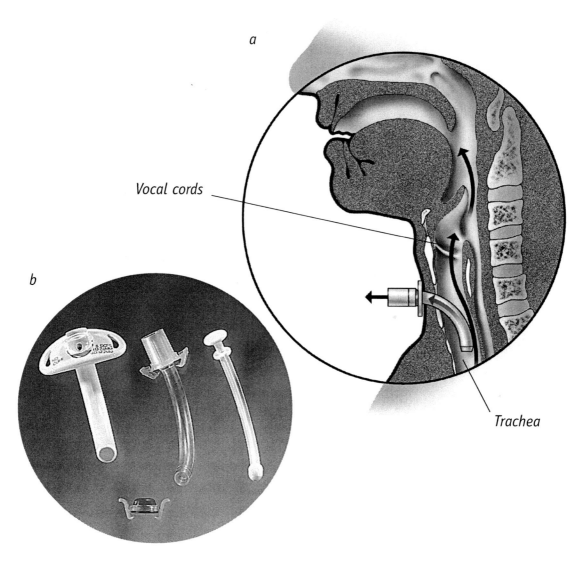

Figure 3.18. A cuffless unfenestrated tracheostomy tube: (a) in situ showing placement and airflow; and (b) components. (Reprinted by permission of Nellcor Puritan Bennett, Inc., Pleasanton, CA.)

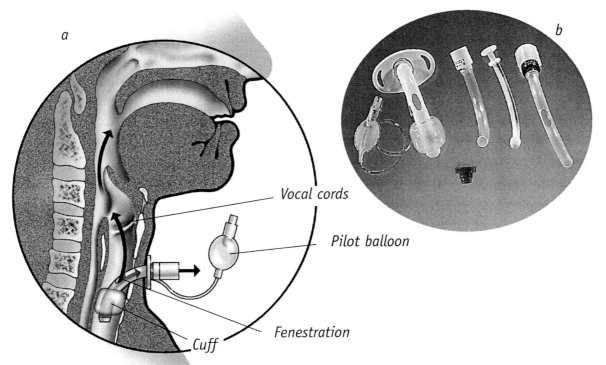

Figure 3.19. A cuffed fenestrated tracheostomy tube: (a) in situ showing placement and airflow; and (b) components. (Reprinted by permission of Nellcor Puritan Bennett, Inc., Pleasanton, CA.)

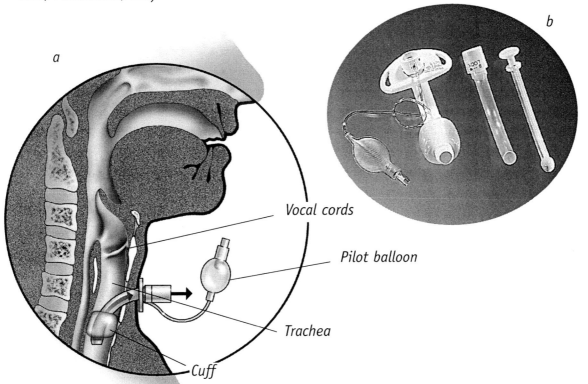

Figure 3.20. A cuffed unfenestrated tracheostomy tube: (a) in situ showing placement and airflow; and (b) components. (Reprinted by permission of Nellcor Puritan Bennett, Inc., Pleasanton, CA.)

▪ Fenestrated Versus Unfenestrated

Recall that fenestrations are openings in the shaft of the inner and outer cannulas. Fenestrated tubes are designed to permit better airflow through the larynx (see figures 3.17 and 3.19, pages 45 and 46). One drawback we have encountered with a fenestrated tube is that tracheal tissue may be pulled, or may grow, into the fenestrations, which increases the risk of developing granuloma tissue. Over time, the granuloma may block the fenestrations, diminishing their effectiveness and complicating the insertion and removal of the inner cannula (see figure 3.21).

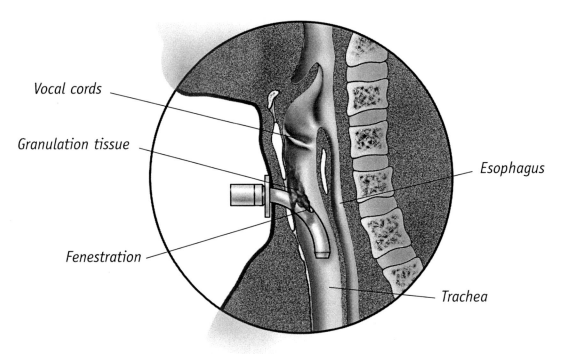

Vocal cords

Granulation tissue

Esophagus

Fenestration

Trachea

Figure 3.21. Granulation tissue partially obstructing the fenestrations of a tracheostomy tube.

▪ Silicone Versus Metal

A tracheostomy tube may be made of either silicone or metal (see figure 3.22). The choice of which to use is often dictated by physician preference and the need for mechanical ventilation. Because a metal tube is cuffless and has a low-profile hub, it cannot be used with a ventilator and requires a special type of speaking valve. It is preferred for relatively long-term tracheostomy needs, in part because tracheal tissue is less likely to adhere to the tube. Silicone tubes are the most widely used, because individuals typically require mechanical ventilation during the onset of respiratory failure.

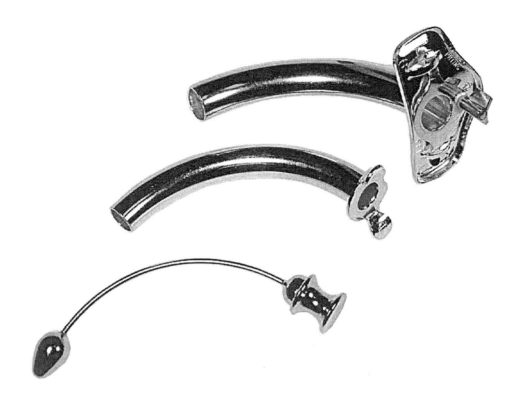

Figure 3.22. Jackson metal tracheostomy tube. (Courtesy of Pilling Surgical)

■ Pediatric Versus Adult Sizes

Due to the variety of shapes and sizes of human airways, tracheostomy tubes come in a range of sizes (see figure 3.23, page 50). Imagine the differences between the airway of a neonate weighing less than three pounds and that of a 250-pound adult. The cannula on the adult-sized tracheostomy tube will most likely be as big as the baby's tiny arm! Neonatal and pediatric tracheostomy tubes typically are cuffless due to the rapid growth and development of the infant's airway and the greater fragility of the tissues. Cuffed pediatric and neonatal tracheostomy tubes may be specially ordered from the manufacturer, however. As a general rule of thumb, a neonatal tracheostomy tube typically fits babies from birth to eighteen months of age; pediatric tracheostomy tubes fit children from one to eight or ten years of age; and a small adult tracheostomy tube will fit most children older than age ten. Everyone is different, and airway size is a more important criterion than age when a physician is determining which tube size to use.

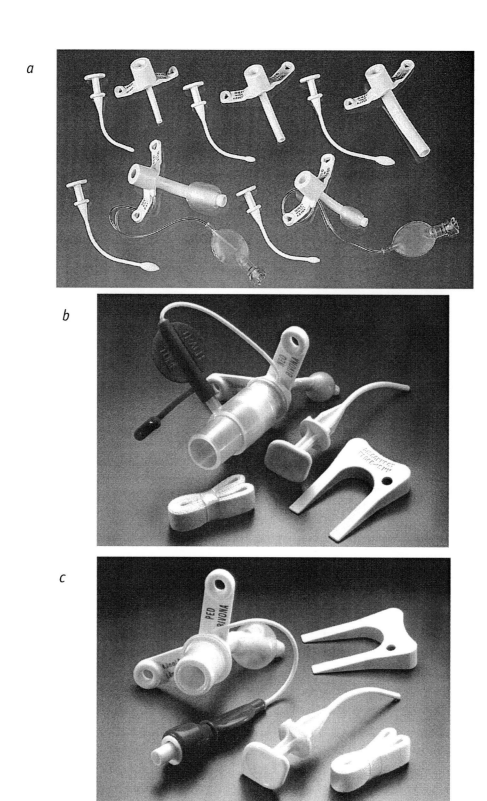

Figure 3.23. (a) Shiley® neonate and pediatric tracheostomy tubes (Reprinted by permission of Nellcor Puritan Bennett, Inc., Pleasanton, CA.); (b) Bivona Fome-Cuf® neonate tracheostomy tube (Courtesy of Bivona Medical Technologies); and (c) Bivona Aire-Cuf® pediatric tracheostomy tube (Courtesy of Bivona Medical Technologies).

■ Talking Versus Non-Talking

Talking tracheostomy tubes, those that facilitate speech despite cuff inflation, will be discussed in more detail in chapter 4. These are a specialized type of tube considered for patients who are candidates for vocal communication but cannot tolerate having the cuff of the tracheostomy tube deflated while speaking. The standard type of tracheostomy tube described thus far is referred to as a non-talking type because it requires a special speaking valve to permit vocal communication.

Conclusion

There are a variety of ways to maintain a patent airway, depending whether the need is temporary or long-term. For temporary circumstances, oral or nasal intubation via an endotracheal tube is preferred. Because this tube passes through the vocal cords, speech and swallowing are impossible while it is in place. For long-term airway management, a tracheostomy tube is inserted into the trachea below the larynx. By becoming familiar with the different types of intubation, especially the implications of their placements, and the parts and characteristics of various tubes, speech-language pathologists are able to make recommendations regarding communication and swallowing while promoting a patient's independence, quality of life and recovery.

Chapter 4
Methods of Communication

The ability to communicate is very powerful. What happens to a person when that ability is suddenly taken away, especially at a time of a dramatic life change when the support of family and friends is needed? The placement of an alternative airway suddenly changes a patient's means of breathing and takes away the ability to speak. Speech-language pathologists have been working to improve, clarify, augment and find alternative means of communication since the beginning of the profession. Working with patients who are tracheostomy- or ventilator-dependent adds a new challenge to the ingenuity of the speech-language pathologist.

To understand why an alternative airway interferes with vocal communication, recall the anatomical placement of endotracheal (ET) and tracheostomy tubes. Whether placed through the nose or mouth, an ET tube passes through the glottis (between the vocal cords) into the trachea (see figure 4.1a, page 54). Thus, the vocal cords are forced open and are unable to approximate or vibrate effectively, eliminating the ability to vocalize. Tracheostomy tubes, on the other hand, are inserted into the trachea between the cartilaginous rings below the cricoid and thyroid cartilages, and thus, below the level of the vocal cords (see figure 4.1b, page 54). Because air now flows in and out through the tracheostomy tube instead of the nose and mouth, there is little, if any, airflow past the vocal cords to create phonation. At times a person is able to phonate if air is forced around the tracheostomy tube, either intentionally or due to an air leak around the inflated cuff. Such forcing of air is discouraged, however, as it puts a great deal of force and pressure against the vocal cords and tracheal walls and tends to force the false vocal folds to vibrate in compensation.

Communication does not require vocalization, however. It can be achieved through gestures, written language, pointing to or looking at pictures or words, and electronic alternative communication devices. Patients who are tracheostomized or ventilator-dependent may utilize multiple means of communication in the interim until vocal communication can be achieved. All means of communication must be explored; every opportunity for communication must be given in an effort to restore that fundamental connection and allow these individuals to communicate their needs and wants. In this chapter, we will begin by describing nonvocal communication options, then move to options such as talking tracheostomy tubes and speaking valves that enable vocal communication.

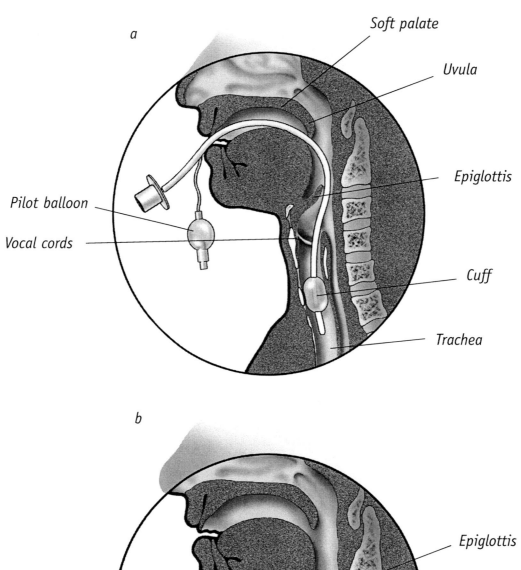

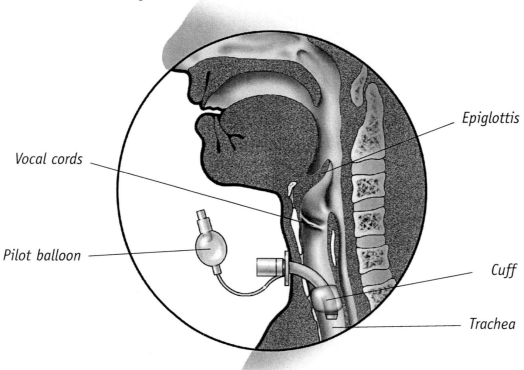

Figure 4.1. Lateral view of oral endotracheal and tracheostomy tube placements: (a) cuffed oral endotracheal tube; (b) cuffed tracheostomy tube placement.

Nonvocal Communication Options

Although vocal communication is typically the desired outcome, communication can be achieved through other means. Patients who are not able to vocalize, especially those who are intubated with an endotracheal tube, should be assessed for an alternative form of communication. Some forms are easily established, others are not. The ultimate goal, however, is to achieve effective and functional communication.

There are two basic forms of augmentative communication, scanning and direct selection. In direct selection, the user chooses the desired response independently (for example, by pointing to a picture), which is the most efficient means. Users who do not have the fine motor ability for direct selection may be able to use a scanning system, in which the listener reads each response in turn, and the patient indicates when the desired response is read. (There are also electronic scanning devices.) Even a patient who is immobilized, for example in a back or neck brace following spinal cord injury, should be able to manage a simple yes/no or scanning system if sufficiently alert.

Very basic communication can be achieved through eye blinks or head nods for yes and no. If a clear plastic board with words written on it is mounted in the patient's visual field, he or she may be able to look at the desired response. Often topics can be written on the board (for example, Needs, Family, What's happening?) to cue the listener to ask questions about that topic. Listeners always need instruction in how to communicate with an alternative communication user, but if a patient has a limited system like this, listener training is especially important. For example, a user of a yes/no system cannot answer, "How are you feeling?" but can respond to "Are you in pain?" "Are you cold?" and so on. It may be helpful to post written instructions or question sequences at bedside to help listeners interact with the patient as efficiently as possible.

For patients who are able, pointing to pictures, letters or words can be an efficient means of communication. Simple, clinician-made communication boards or folders are an inexpensive means of giving the patient at least a limited vocabulary. However, this form of communication has four drawbacks. First, the patient must have enough fine motor control to point with intent and accuracy. When many choices are placed close together on the board, it may be difficult for the patient to isolate the specific selection. Second, the patient must have the cognitive and visual skills to scan the entire board; comprehend the meaning and consequences of each symbol, word or combination of letters to spell; and initiate the effort to communicate (organizing the selections in categories is helpful). Some patients do not have the cognitive alertness to accurately select from a variety of responses. It may be necessary to begin with a simple yes/no and train listeners to ask yes/no questions. This leads to the third and fourth drawbacks: the patient is limited to the options available on the communication system. Frequently the patient may wish to communicate something that is not among the available choices. As well, if the communication system is not where the patient can access it, communication is impossible. It is very important to train family and staff to keep the communication board close to the patient in order for it to be functional and effective.

Electronic communication systems, also referred to as alternative and augmentative devices (AAC devices), can be an option if the technology is available. Sometimes simple four-cell devices (see figure 4.2), into which four statements (or questions) of need or want can be recorded for later playback, may be effective for patients with limited abilities. Options such as "I need to go to the bathroom," "I am hungry or thirsty," "I am in pain," "Where is my family?" can at least allow patients to express basic needs. There is a wide range of complexity in electronic AAC systems, and some will enable extended conversation and increased control over the environment. With the simpler and smaller devices, patients are limited to the choices available. In addition, some motoric means of activation must be established, an area where consultation with occupational or physical therapists is very helpful. Complex devices require high-level cognitive abilities and these devices can be very expensive. However, if this is the best means of communication available to the patient, every effort should be made to identify and obtain the most effective device. (See the vendor list in Appendix B for various AAC device companies.) For some patients, the decision to purchase an expensive electronic AAC device is made after all other options have failed.

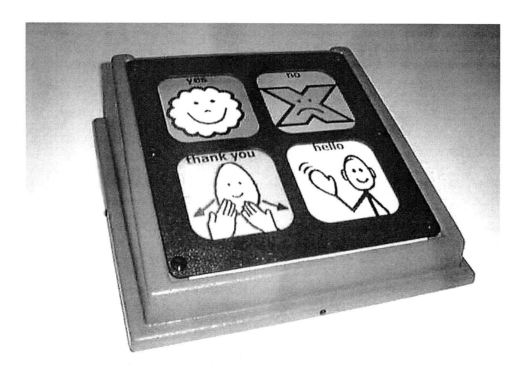

Figure 4.2. Four-cell augmentative communication device. (Courtesy of AMDI)

Writing can also be an effective means of communication if the patient has the motor and cognitive skills to write legibly. (It is always wise to verify that the patient and family are sufficiently literate to use such a system.) Again, writing utensils must be kept within reach of the patient or the means to communicate is lost. Patients who are not able to write may be able to spell out words or phrases by pointing to letters on a small grease board. Sign language or gestures may be another effective means of communication. The two main drawbacks to the use of sign language are that the individual must have the cognitive skills to learn and remember the signs or to develop a gesture system, and the listener must also understand what the signs or gestures mean.

With individuals who will require long-term tracheostomy—especially children who are tracheostomized early in the course of their language development—establishing alternative means of communication is absolutely critical. A child who is not a candidate for the vocal options discussed later in this chapter must be given the opportunity to create a foundation for verbal language, if not vocal language. The use of sign language or augmentative communication will allow these children to learn the language skills they need in order to learn and talk about their world. If later in life the child becomes a candidate for vocal communication, the transition to vocal communication will be easier and more rapid because the child already has developed a foundation of language skills.

Vocal Communication Options

Vocal communication feels more natural, more efficient and more comforting to most individuals, especially those who were able to talk prior to intubation, and most have a strong desire to speak again. Unfortunately, there is no means for patients with an ET tube to communicate vocally until the ET tube is removed. And as will be discussed later in this chapter, even after extubation, vocal communication may be limited or even ineffective. A nonvocal means of alternative communication must be established for these patients. Thus, this section on vocal communication is applicable only for patients who have a tracheostomy tube. There are three ways to facilitate vocalization in a person who has a tracheostomy tube: (a) recommend the use of a talking tracheostomy tube; (b) attempt "leak speech," in which the cuff is partially deflated to permit airflow around the outside of the tube and upward to the larynx; or (c) use a one-way speaking valve.

▣ Talking Tracheostomy Tubes

A talking tracheostomy tube is a specialized type of cuffed tracheostomy tube that has an additional line for airflow. This airflow line terminates just above the cuff, allowing for airflow up into the larynx, between the true vocal cords, and out the mouth and nose. The line is used as an air source for vocalization only and has a port that must be manually occluded to direct airflow from an external air source through the line when the patient wishes to speak (see figure 4.3). Oxygenated air required to maintain adequate ventilation continues to flow through the main tracheostomy tube. The use of talking tracheostomy tubes can be beneficial for those patients who must have the cuff inflated at all times, either because of the need for mechanical ventilation (to be discussed in chapter 6) or because of a significant risk of aspiration (discussed in chapter 5). The talking tracheostomy tube is most appropriate for older children or adults who have the capability to occlude the port when they wish to speak. The change from a traditional tracheostomy tube to the talking tracheostomy tube must be ordered and changed by a healthcare provider.

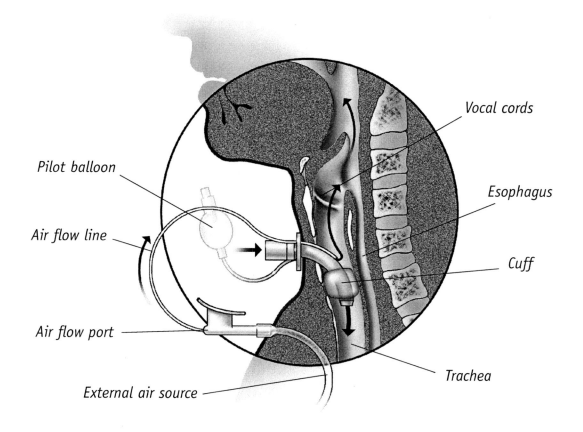

Figure 4.3. Illustration of a talking tracheostomy tube system.

Two brands of talking tracheostomy tubes are available as of 2001, although new products are continually being developed (see figure 4.4). The Portex Trach Talk and the Bivona Talk Trach function as described above. As with the traditional Bivona Fome-Cuf® tracheostomy tube, the Bivona Talk Trach has a foam-filled cuff and does not have an inner cannula. In addition, the talking tube model has a smaller cuff around the stoma to seal it so the supplementary air for vocalization does not leak around the stoma. This secondary cuff is also foam-filled.

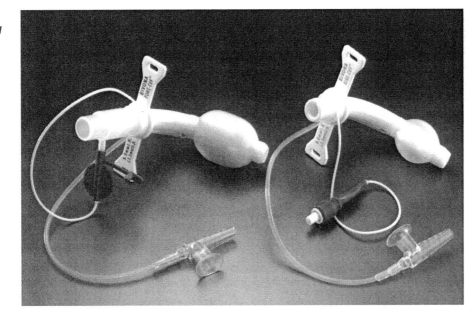

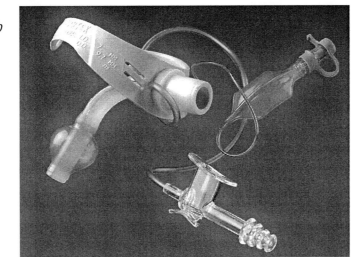

Figure 4.4. (a) Bivona Fome-Cuf® and Aire-Cuf® talking tracheostomy tubes (Courtesy of Bivona Medical Technologies); and (b) Portex Trach Talk talking tracheostomy tube (Courtesy of Portex, Inc.).

To be a candidate for the talking tracheostomy tube, a patient must meet the following criteria.

1. The upper airway must be free of occlusions or stenoses so that adequate airflow can pass through the vocal cords for phonation and out through the mouth for articulation.

2. The vocal cords must be functional to produce adequate phonation for speech.

3. The patient is unable to tolerate cuff deflation for other forms of vocal communication (such as a speaking valve to be discussed later in this chapter).

4. The patient should not have a neuromuscular disease. The literature documents

limited success with such patients because of their difficulty coordinating the articulators (Gordon 1984).

5. The patient must not have excessive saliva production or oral secretions. The buildup of saliva or aspiration of oral secretions and phlegm eventually will occlude the airflow line.

6. It is preferable, although not always necessary, for the patient to have the motor skills to occlude the airflow port independently when he or she wishes to speak. (Family members can be trained to occlude the port, but this greatly lessens the patient's ability to communicate independently.)

A thorough chart review will often indicate whether a patient meets these criteria. Documentation of tracheomalacia, pharyngeal stenosis, subglottic stenosis, pharyngeal growths or tumors, or similar diagnoses is likely to disqualify the patient. Other red flags include emergent intubation of an endotracheal tube, multiple extubations and reintubations of endotracheal tubes, or multiple episodes of aspiration. (Emergent or repeated placement and removal of an ET tube can lead to vocal cord damage from the tube being repeatedly forced between the vocal cords. Multiple episodes of aspiration may indicate vocal cord dysfunction.) If there is any question about the condition of the airway, the patient should be referred to an otolaryngologist for an assessment of upper airway patency and adequate vocal cord function prior to the insertion of a talking tracheostomy tube.

Clinical trials with the talking tracheostomy tube typically begin forty-eight to seventy-two hours after insertion, to allow the surrounding tissues to heal and the swelling to diminish. An external air supply (either a compressed air or an oxygen canister) must be attached to the airflow port. Once the air source is connected, begin the flow at three to five liters per minute (lpm). Have the patient (or a caregiver) use a finger to occlude the port, directing airflow into the trachea, while cueing the individual to attempt to vocalize. Gradually increase the rate of flow from the external source until the patient's speech is audible and intelligible. (This typically occurs at a flow rate of eight liters per minute or greater.) As the rate of airflow increases, the patient may experience discomfort from the dry air passing over the vocal cords and the pressure being exerted on the larynx, so it is preferable to maintain the airflow below fifteen liters per minute. Although it would be preferable to humidify the supplemental air, it is difficult to humidify air through such a narrow tube.

Talking tracheostomy tubes have some disadvantages. They are more expensive than standard tracheostomy tubes, and the cost of the supplemental air source also must be considered. One of the most common problems is a buildup of secretions above the cuff, blocking off or limiting the airflow for speech. Each manufacturer has specific guidelines for how to reduce or clear away these secretions, and these guidelines should be followed. It is possible to suction through the airflow line, but doing so creates risks of either collapsing the tubing or drawing a plug of secretions into the line, both of which would significantly reduce or eliminate the airflow through it.

Leak Speech

Leak speech is used to describe phonation achieved by air leaking around a partially deflated cuff. Usually the cuff is purposely deflated for speaking valve trials, but sometimes a patient will force air around an inflated cuff in an effort to speak. (As mentioned previously, doing so should be discouraged because of the potential to damage tracheal tissue.) Leak speech is a useful option for patients who cannot tolerate full cuff deflation due to a high aspiration risk or inability to tolerate pressure or airflow changes in the pharynx. Candidates for leak speech must have strong enough respiratory support to produce sufficient airflow through the larynx for audible phonation. This method of communication is most often used on a temporary basis and may be used for preliminary trials of vocal ability. If the individual is able to vocalize using leak speech, however, steps should be taken to increase tolerance of full cuff deflation for use of a one-way speaking valve. The use of a speaking valve is preferable to leak speech because of the improvements in swallowing ability that often result (see chapter 5).

One-Way Speaking Valves

A one-way speaking valve provides another means of directing airflow through the vocal cords to allow phonation. This type of valve allows air to be inhaled through the tracheostomy tube, but it closes on exhalation so that the air is exhaled around the outside of rather than through the tracheostomy tube. To be a candidate for such a valve the patient *must* be able to tolerate having the cuff fully deflated. Recall that an inflated cuff completely blocks the trachea, and since the valve prevents air from escaping through the tracheostomy tube, the patient would have no way to exhale. For this reason, the Bivona Fome-Cuf® foam-filled cuffed tracheostomy tube is *not compatible* with a speaking valve as its foam-filled cuff tends to self-inflate over time. If an individual with a Bivona Fome-Cuf® tracheostomy tube demonstrates tolerance of cuff deflation, recommend to the physician that the tracheostomy tube be changed to one with an air-filled cuff in order to allow speaking valve trials. As will be discussed in chapter 6, only the group of Passy-Muir Speaking Valves are designed for use with a mechanical ventilator.

The one-way speaking valve has many advantages. Not only does it facilitate speech, it increases pharyngeal sensation and awareness, improves the senses of taste and smell, can decrease the volume of secretions and facilitates a safer swallow. With airflow restored up into the larynx and above, pharyngeal sensation is increased and the senses of taste and smell are improved. Heightened sensation may cue patients to swallow their own secretions, and the restored airflow may result in decreased secretions. Without the speaking valve, it is very hard to close off the glottis to protect the airway, since there is very little air with which to create the necessary subglottic pressure to adduct the vocal cords. With the speaking valve, air flows into the larynx and enough pressure can be created to protect the airway effectively, facilitating a safer swallow. The patient may also be better able to sense penetration or aspiration and initiate a cough. Coughing is typically stronger with a speaking valve than without because of the increased ability to create subglottic pressure.

The speaking valve attaches to the hub of the inner cannula (see figure 4.5). Most speaking valves have a thin membrane or diaphragm that allows air to flow into the tracheostomy tube during inhalation but closes off during exhalation. Many brands of speaking valves are available. The Shiley® Phonate Speaking Valve, Passy-Muir Speaking Valve and Montgomery® Speaking Valve models fit the standard-sized fifteen-millimeter hub on a plastic tracheostomy tube. Because metal tubes are a different size and have a low-profile hub, they require valves specifically designed to fit them. (Some manufacturers have an inner cannula with a fifteen-millimeter hub that can be specially ordered if needed, but this is not always the most practical or cost-effective solution.) The speaking valves available for metal tracheostomy tubes are the Kistner Valve, the Passy-Muir Speaking Valve 2020 and the Tucker Valve. Originally designed to fit the Jackson metal tracheostomy tube, the Shikani-French valve is now available in two models, one for metal and the other for plastic tracheostomy tubes.

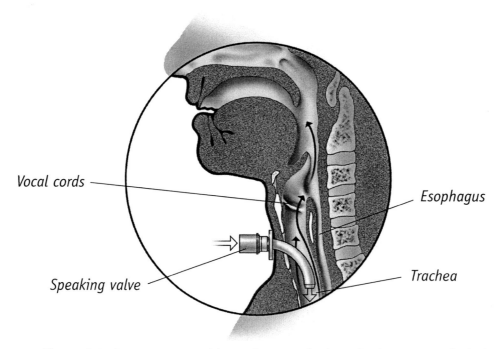

Figure 4.5. A one-way speaking valve attached to the inner cannula hub.

Speaking Valves for Plastic Tracheostomy Tubes

One-way speaking valves commonly used with plastic tracheostomy tubes include the Shiley® Phonate Speaking Valve, the Montgomery® Speaking Valve, and a "family" of Passy-Muir Speaking Valves. These models fit the Shiley,® Portex or Bivona Aire-Cuf® plastic tracheostomy tubes. Here is how these valves differ:

The Shiley® Phonate has two unique features, a "flip top" that allows for easier cleaning and suctioning, and one model that has an oxygen port attached to the speaking valve for direct oxygenation (see figure 4.6). One disadvantage is that oxygen tubing attached to the oxygen port of the Shiley® Phonate can cause unwanted tugging on the tracheostomy tube if the patient is not careful to keep enough slack available.

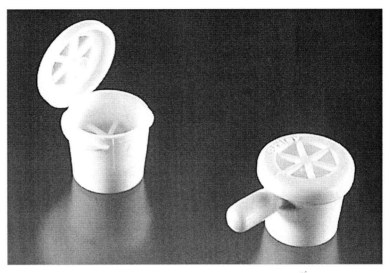

Figure 4.6. Shiley® Phonate speaking valve. (Reprinted by permission of Nellcor Puritan Bennett, Inc., Pleasanton, CA.)

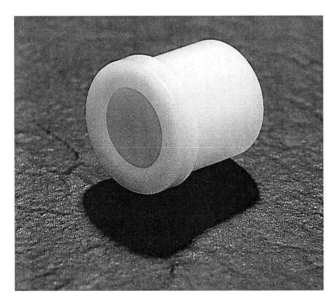

Figure 4.7. Montgomery® speaking valve. (Courtesy of Boston Medical Technologies)

The Montgomery® Speaking Valve is unique for its pressure-release feature (see figure 4.7). Should the patient cough hard enough to potentially dislodge the speaking valve from the hub, the diaphragm will detach and blow out through the casing of the valve, preventing the entire valve from coming off. The obvious advantage is that the speaking valve does not have to be cleaned and replaced repeatedly whenever the patient coughs, but there are disadvantages as well. Repeatedly having to reinsert the diaphragm in the casing increases the risk of damage. Over time the diaphragm also tends to loosen in the casing until it can be dislodged during even minor coughing spells.

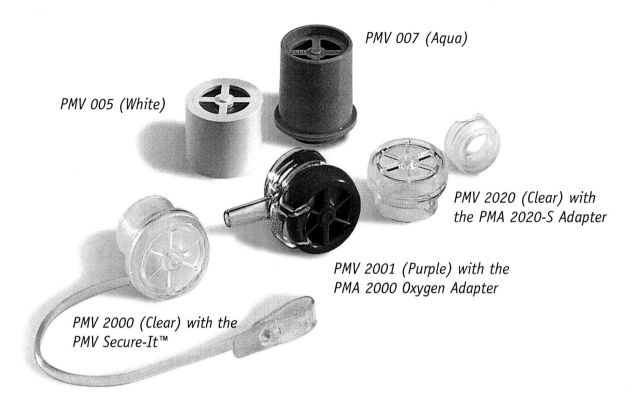

PMV 005 (White)

PMV 007 (Aqua)

PMV 2020 (Clear) with
the PMA 2020-S Adapter

PMV 2001 (Purple) with the
PMA 2000 Oxygen Adapter

PMV 2000 (Clear) with the
PMV Secure-It™

Figure 4.8. Variety of Passy-Muir speaking valves. (Photo courtesy of Passy-Muir, Inc.)

The Passy-Muir Speaking Valve, or PMV, actually denotes a family of valves (see figure 4.8). These valves are marketed as the only valves with a "closed-position, no-leak" design, meaning that at rest the valve remains closed, opening with minimal resistance only during inspiration. The manufacturer provides research documentation for the advantages to this design (Passy-Muir 1999). First, since the PMV remains in a closed position except during inhalation, a column of air is trapped inside the tracheostomy tube, resisting the collection of secretions inside the tracheostomy tube and the PMV. Second, the valve reduces the effort of breathing since the patient must exert energy only to open the valve. In contrast, valves that remain in the open position at rest require effort to open and close the valve with every breath. (Although the amount of effort required is minimal in theory, some patients with a weak respiratory system and multiple medical complications fatigue with use of a speaking valve and may need to build up their endurance before they can wear it for extended periods of time.) Finally, unlike open-position valves, the PMV has been documented to improve swallowing function. The Passy-Muir Speaking Valves are also the only valves that can be used in-line with a ventilator (see chapter 6 for protocols). The PMV 007 (the aqua-colored valve), can be used in-line with a ventilator if disposable tubing is used. The PMV 005 (white), 2000 (clear) and 2001 (purple) valves can be used in-line with a ventilator if non-disposable tubing is used.

Methods of Communication

Speaking Valves for Metal Tracheostomy Tubes

The Kistner Valve is unique in that it twists on and locks into place on the low-profile hub. The locking mechanism may be a concern if the valve must be removed quickly during an episode of respiratory distress. Because of the locking feature, the entire tracheostomy tube may inadvertently be pulled out, instead of just the valve. Accidental removal of the tracheostomy tube is a significant problem that can lead to respiratory failure.

The Shikani-French valve is a new design using a ball-and-hole mechanism (see figure 4.9). Instead of a membranous valve, there is a hole at the front of the valve and a small ball that fits into the hole far enough to occlude it. During inhalation the ball is drawn away from the hole, but during exhalation the outgoing airflow forces the ball into the hole, preventing any further air loss through the valve. This design means that operation of the valve is affected by position: a recumbent patient must use more effort to close the valve than a patient who is upright. Although we have not used this valve extensively, in initial trials we have found it very difficult to remove in case of respiratory distress, placing the patient at risk for accidental extubation (removal of the tracheostomy tube) during the attempt to remove the valve. It is possible that with extended use, the mechanism may loosen up enough to make placement and removal of the valve easier.

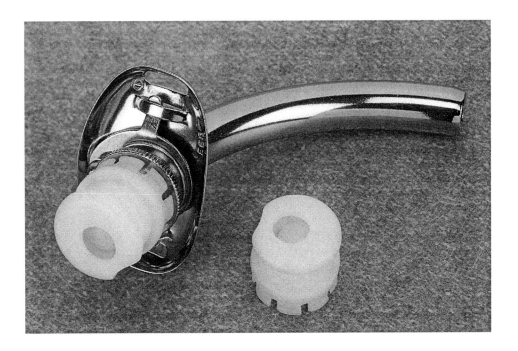

Figure 4.9. Shikani-French speaking valve on a metal tracheostomy tube. (A model that fits plastic tracheostomy tubes is available but not pictured.) (Courtesy of Pilling Surgical)

The Passy-Muir Speaking Valve 2020 (PMV 2020) is a new product which, when used with the Passy-Muir PMA 2020-S adapter, fits the Pilling Weck Improved Jackson tracheostomy tube (see figure 4.8, page 64). The PMV 2020 valve uses a membrane and functions in the same way as the other Passy-Muir valves described previously. Bear in mind that the PMV 2020 cannot be used in-line because all Jackson tracheostomy tubes are incompatible with ventilators. Any of the Passy-Muir Speaking Valves (which are usually attached to plastic tracheostomy tubes) can be attached to a metal tracheostomy tube in one of two ways: a fifteen-millimeter hub can be specially ordered from the manufacturer, or an endotracheal tube adapter can be sized to fit the low-profile metal tracheostomy tube, creating a fifteen-millimeter hub for attachment.

The Tucker Valve is not a free-standing valve as the other one-way speaking valves are. Instead it is integrated into the tracheostomy tube itself (see figure 4.10). The Tucker Valve fits like a trap door over a fenestration on the inner cannula of a fenestrated Jackson tracheostomy tube. The valve rests tip-down inside the inner cannula. During inhalation through the tracheostomy tube, the valve is forced up to occlude the fenestration. During exhalation the tip drops, redirecting the air through the fenestration and up to the larynx.

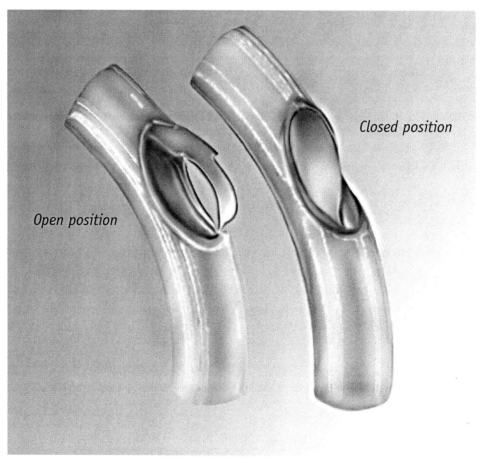

Figure 4.10. Tucker Valve. (Courtesy of Pilling Surgical)

Candidacy for a Speaking Valve

To be a candidate for a speaking valve, a patient must meet the following criteria:

1. The upper airway must be free of obstructions or stenoses so that air can flow freely through the vocal cords for phonation and through the mouth for articulation.

2. The patient must be able to tolerate cuff deflation.

3. The vocal cords must be functional to produce adequate phonation for speech. A preliminary screening for vocal cord function and speaking valve tolerance can be done by deflating the cuff, placing a gloved finger over the end of the tracheostomy tube and asking the patient to vocalize. (As will be discussed later, sometimes the integrity of the vocal cords cannot be determined until a trial with a one-way speaking valve.)

4. The patient must not be using the Bivona Fome-Cuf® tracheostomy tube. If the patient currently has this type of tube, ask the physician about the possibility of changing the tracheostomy tube to another brand to enable vocal communication.

5. If patient has excessive amounts of secretions, management of the secretions should be addressed before a speaking valve is inserted. Although the use of a one-way speaking valve may reduce the amount of secretions, a patient who has thick secretions may not be a good candidate for a speaking valve.

6. The patient should be medically stable and should not have other pressing medical needs or complications.

Use of a Fenestrated Tracheostomy Tube with a Speaking Valve

There has been a fair amount of discussion regarding the need for a fenestrated tracheostomy tube with a speaking valve. Although many physicians were trained that a fenestrated tracheostomy tube is required for vocal communication, we have not found this necessarily to be the case. On the contrary, in our practice we have discovered that the fenestrations seem to promote the growth of granulation tissue, which grows into the fenestrations and occludes them. We have also found that a one-way speaking valve can be used with both fenestrated and unfenestrated types of tracheostomy tubes (excluding the Bivona Fome-Cuf®), and speaking trials can be initiated as early as forty-eight to seventy-two hours after the initial intubation or twelve to twenty-four hours after a tracheostomy tube change. (These time frames may vary depending on the amount of trauma to and swelling of the tissues surrounding the tracheostomy tube.)

If the patient does already have a fenestrated tracheostomy tube, it is not usually necessary to request a tracheostomy tube change. Following the protocol for speaking valve use given later in this chapter, try the speaking valve with the fenestrated inner cannula. If that inner cannula has been lost, as happens quite frequently, try the following suggestions to accommodate the speaking valve. First, try a regular, unfenestrated inner cannula. Whether this will work depends on the relative diameters of the tracheostomy tube and the airway; if the tube is sized such that minimal air can flow around the outside, the use of an unfenestrated inner cannula will not be effective. In this case, take a sterile unfenestrated inner cannula and cut off the distal end just before the bend, about one inch beyond the hub and just past the size number embossed into it. This "clipped" inner cannula allows air to flow out the fenestrations in the outer cannula while still providing a hub on which to attach the speaking valve (see figure 4.11, page 69). Be sure, however, to remove the clipped inner cannula when the speaking valve is removed and to replace it with a clean inner cannula. Clean and store the clipped inner cannula with the valve for future use.

■ Caution about Patients with a Laryngectomy

It is vital to recognize the difference between a metal tracheostomy tube and a metal laryngectomy tube used post-surgery. Patients who have undergone a laryngectomy sometimes require a temporary means of preventing the stoma from closing post-surgery. Either a tracheostomy tube or special metal laryngectomy tube may be used for this purpose. Attempting to place a speaking valve on a laryngectomy tube is very dangerous and should never be attempted. The valve will render the patient unable to exhale, resulting in suffocation. Moreover, laryngectomy removes the entire larynx, including the vocal cords, so a speaking valve is ineffective and inappropriate for these patients. Never attempt to place a speaking valve on any patient who has undergone a laryngectomy.

Clinical Trials of a Speaking Valve

The following is a protocol for initiating clinical trials once the patient is determined to be a candidate for speaking valve use. (See page 67 for candidacy criteria.) Use your clinical judgment to adjust these steps as necessary, depending on how well the patient tolerates the valve and what resources are available at the time of the trial. In our practice, we have found that having a respiratory therapist present for at least the initial trials is very helpful, particularly for clinicians who are inexperienced with patients who have speaking valves. Working as a team, the respiratory therapist can monitor the respiratory function of the patient while you focus on speech production. Once the patient's tolerance for the valve has been determined and you feel confident in your ability to handle any respiratory difficulty the individual may have, it is possible to do further treatment sessions without the respiratory therapist present. In contrast, the use of a speaking valve in-line with a ventilator almost always necessitates a respiratory therapist or nurse trained in ventilator management to make

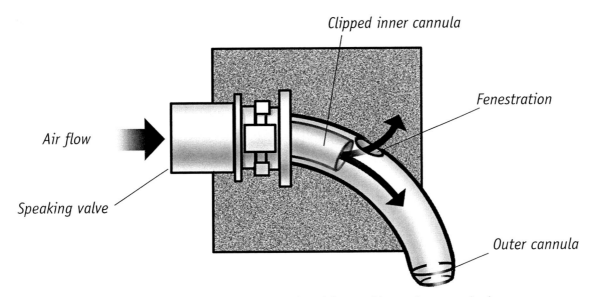

Clipped inner cannula

Fenestration

Air flow

Speaking valve

Outer cannula

Figure 4.11. Clipped inner cannula with speaking valve attached.

the required changes to the ventilator settings.

Before clinical trials can begin, baseline measurements of oxygen saturation percentage, resting heart rate, breathing rate, effort required for breathing, coloring and level of anxiety must be taken. (The procedures for taking these measures, and their expected ranges, begin on page 25.) It is also helpful to note the positioning of the patient, whether upright at a 90-degree angle, reclined at a 45-degree angle or sidelying. These measures are repeated after placement and again after removal of the valve. If a patient is unable to maintain or recover quickly to near baseline levels when using a speaking valve, its use should be discontinued. A reproducible form for monitoring the patient's status throughout the trial is provided on page 70.

■ Protocol for Clinical Trials of the Speaking Valve

1. Take baseline measurements of oxygen saturation percentage, heart rate, respiratory rate, effort of breathing, and position.

2. If the tracheostomy tube has a cuff, deflate it. Be sure to measure carefully how much air you withdraw so you can reinflate the cuff to the proper level after the trial. (Mark baseline measures at the initiation of the first trial of cuff deflation.)

3. Encourage the patient to cough or clear his or her throat as needed. Suction the patient's trachea and mouth, if secretions are present.

4. Attach the speaking valve to the tracheostomy tube according to the manufacturer's instructions and record the time the trial begins. Reassure the patient that it is normal for breathing to feel different with the valve in place, and monitor the individual for anxiety.

5. Suction orally if needed; encourage the patient to cough and clear his or her throat as needed to mobilize loose secretions.

Speaking Valve Trial Flow Sheet

Patient:

Patient ID:

Date:

Trach type/size: [ ] Cuff   [ ] No cuff   [ ] Fenestrated

Valve used:

Oxygen:

Start time:

End time:

1.	Baseline measures	O_2: HR: RR: Color: Effort:
2.	Deflate cuff	Amount of air withdrawn: cc
3.	Suction trachea and oral cavity	Amount/color of secretions: Strength of cough:
4.	Place speaking valve	Time placed:
5.	Suction orally	Secretions:
6.	Repeat measures	O_2: HR: RR: Color: Effort:
7.	Cue voicing	Vocal quality:
8.	Repeat measures	O_2: HR: RR: Color: Effort:
9.	Remove valve	Time removed:
10.	Inflate cuff	Amount of air replaced: cc
11.	Repeat measures	O_2: HR: RR: Color: Effort:

Comments:

Speech pathologist:

Respiratory therapist:

Physician:

Key:

O_2 = oxygen saturation percentage   HR = heart rate   RR = respiratory rate

Color = color of face   Effort = amount of effort required for breathing

6. Repeat the baseline measurements while observing breathing. If the patient demonstrates signs of respiratory distress (see page 71) or significant anxiety, remove the valve, reinflate the cuff and monitor how long it takes the patient to recover to baseline measures.

7. If the patient's respiratory status is at or near baseline levels, ask the person to say something (such as counting to ten or reciting the days of the week).

8. Guide the patient in continued speech practice while monitoring his or her status. Terminate the trial immediately if the patient shows signs of respiratory distress. Otherwise continue until the scheduled end of your session.

9. Remove the speaking valve and record the time of removal.

10. Reinflate the cuff with the exact amount of air withdrawn at the beginning of the trial.

11. Repeat the measures taken at baseline. If they are below baseline levels, continue monitoring to determine how long it takes the patient to recover to baseline measures after valve use.

Once the speaking valve is placed on the tracheostomy tube, it is important to give the patient something to say. A routine task such as counting from one to ten, naming the days of the week or months of the year, or even just vocalizing "aah" will help divert the patient's mind from the change in breathing and focus it on vocalization attempts. Sometimes throat clearing or coughing may help with the initiation of voicing. Once the patient is able to sustain voicing, you may choose to conduct a cognitive screening and to assess vocal quality at this time.

Initial trials of the valve should last only as long as you, a respiratory therapist, or a nurse can remain present because of the risk of respiratory distress. Initial therapeutic trials may last as little as a minute or as long as a few hours. Once the patient has demonstrated consistent tolerance of the speaking valve, it can remain in place as long as the person is awake and is not demonstrating signs of distress. Always remember that patients who are tracheostomized may fluctuate greatly in their skills, endurance and tolerance from day to day, so never leave any patient unattended until you are absolutely sure he or she actually does tolerate the valve consistently. Also teach the patient, family members, and caregivers to recognize signs of distress and fatigue, as well as the proper procedures for placing, removing, caring for, and storing the valve.

■ Recognizing the Signs of Respiratory Distress

As you will recall from chapter 2, respiratory distress refers to the inability to achieve adequate airflow or levels of oxygenation to maintain bodily functions. It is signaled by certain atypical behaviors, which are described in this section. Deflating the cuff of the tracheostomy tube and placing a speaking valve on the hub change the parameters of the airway and may alter the patient's respiratory status. For that reason, it is imperative that measurements of respiratory status be documented before, during and after speaking valve use. Clinical and behavioral signs of respiratory distress include the following.

A steady drop in oxygen saturation without a return to baseline measures. Many patients take a moment or two to adjust to the change in breathing after placement of the speaking valve, and it is not uncommon for saturation levels to drop briefly before rebounding to the baseline level, or close to it. For some patients, the physician has written specific orders to maintain oxygenation levels above a certain percentage (for example, "O_2 to keep sats > 92%"). In such cases if the level of oxygen saturation drops below the ordered percentage for more than a few minutes without showing signs of recovery, use of the valve should be discontinued until it can be determined why the saturations remained depressed. The physician may decide that it is necessary to delay further trials until the patient's overall respiratory status improves. Alternatively, if the patient is receiving supplemental oxygen, the physician may determine that the amount of oxygen can be increased during speaking valve use. Such determination should come directly from the physician and be so documented.

Increases in heart and respiratory rates without a return to baseline levels. Again, a brief increase followed by a return to baseline or near-baseline readings is not uncommon when patients first adjust to the valve. Small increases in heart or breathing rates may be tolerable if the patient does not become fatigued or demonstrate any other signs of distress.

Sweating. Diaphoresis, or intense sweating, is a sign of physiologic distress that indicates the patient is unable to tolerate the speaking valve.

Facial expressions of distress. The patient's eyes may widen and the face show an expression of alarm. Patients who cannot vocalize or are having difficulty breathing can express a great deal through their facial expressions.

Signs of struggle. The patient may start gasping for breath or trying to gulp in air. Patients who are having trouble breathing also often use the accessory muscles in the neck and shoulders in an effort to inspire more air (also described as increased work of breathing). The nares flare out and the intercostal muscles retract. These behavioral signs are also seen in children and babies who are having difficulty breathing.

Complaints of dizziness or lightheadedness. A low level of oxygen in the brain will cause sensations of dizziness or lightheadedness. If a patient reports feeling this way, remove the speaking valve.

Decreased responsiveness. It is very possible for the preceding clinical signs and behaviors to appear normal, including oxygen saturation level and heart rate, when the patient is in fact experiencing respiratory distress. A patient who seems to be losing alertness, starts to "drift away" mentally, or goes from being responsive and following commands to a state of unresponsiveness is very likely in respiratory distress. As part of the respiratory process, a person must exhale carbon dioxide as well as take in oxygen. Patients who are unable to exhale, or blow off, carbon dioxide will become increasingly unresponsive as carbon dioxide builds up in their systems. Should you notice a change in alertness, immediately remove the speaking valve and notify the respiratory therapist, nurse or physician of your concerns and the changes you have observed in the patient. The only way to know for certain whether carbon dioxide levels are elevated is to request an arterial blood gas (ABG) draw during the speaking valve trial.

Troubleshooting Difficulties with the Speaking Valve

There are many possible reasons why a patient may have difficulty tolerating the speaking valve during a given trial. Because many patients' medical conditions fluctuate, it may be wise to conduct another trial on a different day to ensure that the patient was not merely having an "off day." If the difficulty does not appear to be a temporary condition, review Table 4.1 (page 74) for possible causes and solutions.

Using Speaking Valves with Infants and Children

It is easy to forget that infants and children are not miniature adults. They have different psychological needs, rely more heavily on communicative interactions and, as discussed in chapter 1, their anatomy is different from an adult's (see figure 1.5, page 10).

Pediatric Airway Differences Affecting the Use of a Speaking Valve

Children have faster reaction times to changes than do adults. This means that a child can adapt quickly to the changes created by the speaking valve but may also decompensate quickly due to smaller reserves of respiratory function and endurance. It is important to recognize the differences in pediatric anatomy that can influence the use of a speaking valve:

- The soft palate is much larger relative to the oral cavity than is an adult's. This fosters nasal breathing and protection of the nasal cavity from nasal regurgitation during swallowing.

- The mucous membranes that line the child's airway are more loosely attached.

- The child's airway has a larger proportion of soft tissue so the potential for edema and swelling is greater.

- An infant's airway has a smaller lumen and is more rapidly obstructed by swelling.

- An infant's airway is more prone to spasm than is an adult's because the airway

Table 4.1. Possible causes of and solutions to difficulty using a speaking valve

Problem	Possible Causes	Possible Solutions
The patient is unable to exhale efficiently through the mouth and nose and cannot achieve voicing.	• The cuff may still be totally or partially inflated. • There may be an upper airway obstruction (including vocal cord dysfunction). • The tracheostomy tube may be too large to allow airflow around it. • The patient may be holding his or her breath.	• Attempt to deflate the cuff again. • Suction the airway to remove any secretions. • Recommend evaluation for upper airway obstruction, including possible vocal cord paralysis in adducted position. • Request that the physician downsize the tracheostomy tube, if possible. • Guide the patient in exhaling through the mouth and nose. • Provide education to reduce anxiety.
The patient is able to breathe efficiently while wearing the speaking valve but is unable to achieve voicing.	• Vocal cord dysfunction may be present (the vocal folds remain abducted).	• Recommend a flexible bronchoscopy or laryngoscopy to evaluate vocal cord function. • Try vocal cord adduction exercises.
The patient has difficulty breathing efficiently while wearing the speaking valve but can produce forced vocalizations.	• The cuff may be partially inflated. • The upper airway may be partially obstructed (including vocal cord dysfunction). • The tracheostomy tube may be too large to allow adequate airflow around it.	• Attempt to deflate the cuff again. • Request a change to a cuffless tracheostomy tube. • Recommend a flexible bronchoscopy or laryngoscopy to evaluate vocal cord function. • Request that the physician downsize the tracheostomy tube, if possible. • Reposition the patient in as straight and upright a position as possible, making sure that the neck is not flexed.

Tracheostomy Tubes and Ventilator Dependence in Adults and Children—VanDahm and Sparks-Walsh

has less cartilaginous support.

■ Recognizing Respiratory Distress in Infants and Children

All the behavioral signs seen in adults may be seen in infants and children, but there are additional behavioral signs of respiratory distress that are not seen in

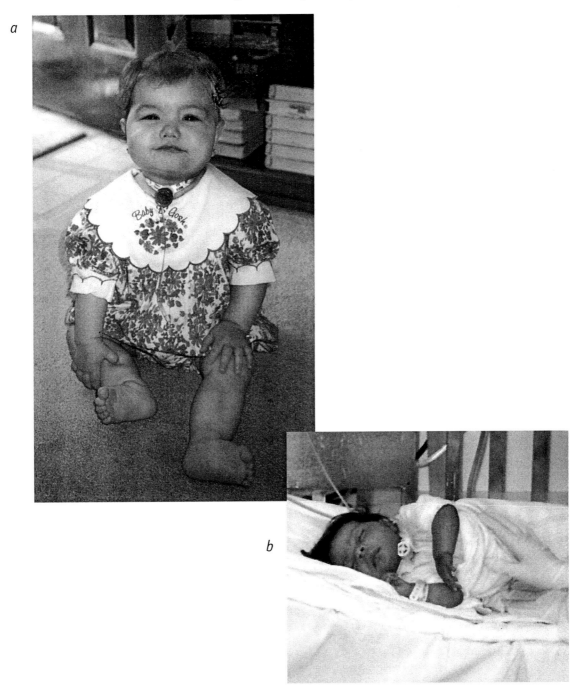

Figure 4.12. (a) Child with PMV; and (b) infant with PMV. (Courtesy of Passy-Muir Inc.)

adults. Because infants and small children are less able to communicate how they are feeling, it is important to watch their behavior carefully. Significant behavioral signs include increased restlessness, increased irritability, grunting (in infants), nasal flaring, head bobbing, neck extension, and paleness or mottling of the skin (a spider web–like network of veins apparent just below the surface of the skin).

◼ Timing of Speaking Valve Trials

Whenever possible (barring medical concerns), initial trials of the speaking valve should occur as soon after tracheostomy tube placement as possible so that the child can acclimate to the changes in both breathing and speech right away. In many cases, however, this is not possible. If there is long delay between tracheostomy tube placement and speaking valve use, early treatment goals may include decreasing anxiety over changes in breathing patterns and familiarizing the child with the valve. Passy-Muir, Inc., markets a stuffed dinosaur with a tracheostomy tube and casings of low-profile Passy-Muir Speaking Valves that young children can explore and learn about. An old tracheostomy tube can also be fitted into a child's own stuffed toy to help the child adjust psychologically. Older children can be taught how to place the speaking valves on their own tracheostomy tubes, as well as how to remove, clean and store them when not in use. It is amazing how many children will learn to deliberately remove the valve to gain attention. This is developmentally appropriate behavior for children, and although not recommended and not tolerated by most parents, it is a means of communication for some children.

Infants who are tracheostomized or ventilator-dependent early in life come to view their tracheostomy or ventilator tubing and equipment as part of their physical identity and personal environment. Infants who are tracheostomized early on in their language development do not develop typical vocal communication skills. Whereas typically developing infants learn the power of the voice and that their cries can gain a response from caregivers, children with a tracheostomy have less ability to vocalize. Instead, they learn how to set off alarms that will evoke a response from caregivers. In addition, the developmental language milestones of cooing and babbling are often missed because of the inability to vocalize consistently and in response to other sounds. The use of speaking valves with infants is vital to the development of their language skills. In fact, two studies have shown that infant tracheostomy may lead to later difficulties with language acquisition, vocal quality and articulation (Kaslon and Stein 1985; Singer et al. 1989). For that reason alone, any infant or child who has a tracheostomy should be considered a candidate for a speaking valve if the requisite criteria is met.

Conclusion

Enabling communication for people who are dependent on tracheostomy tubes is a very critical step in restoring that basic element of their humanity. Evaluation of the type of communication that can be achieved, careful monitoring of the patient and the ability to troubleshoot complications that arise will enable clinicians to re-establish the connection of language. Whether vocal or nonvocal, communication is vitally important for people of all ages. With infants and children whose language development may be disrupted by tracheotomy tube placement, establishing the most effective and efficient possible means to communicate is critical.

Chapter 5
Tracheostomy and Dysphagia

Many individuals who experience serious illness or traumatic injury also experience some form of dysphagia (disorder of swallowing). Because the presence of the tracheostomy tube alters the anatomy of breathing, it is our strong recommendation that all tracheostomized individuals—adults and infants—be evaluated for dysphagia prior to the introduction of food or liquid by mouth. After a brief review of the phases of the normal swallow, this chapter will address the common problems associated with swallowing with a tracheostomy tube and different solutions to overcome these problems.

Phases of the Normal Swallow

It is important to review the basics of swallowing anatomy and function before addressing potential problems of swallowing due to the presence of a tracheostomy tube. Recall that the airway has three levels of protection: the epiglottis, the false vocal folds, and the true vocal cords. The coordinated movement of these structures during a swallow assists in preventing foreign material from entering the airway and potentially causing aspiration pneumonia. The normal swallow occurs in four stages (see figure 5.1, page 80): the oral preparatory phase, the oral transit phase, the pharyngeal phase, and the cervical-esophageal phase.

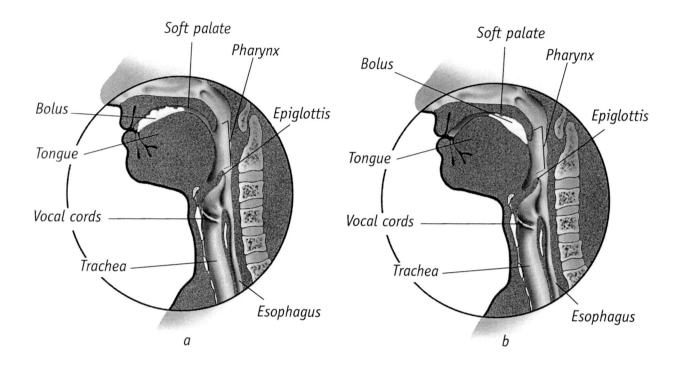

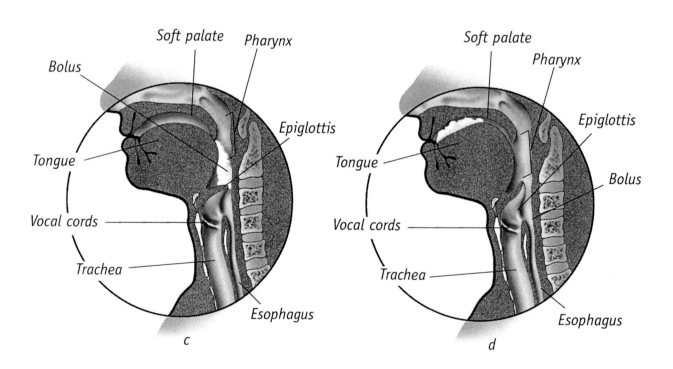

Figure 5.1. Four stages swallowing: (a) oral preparatory; (b) oral transit; (c) pharyngeal; (d) cervical-esophageal.

Oral preparatory phase. The oral preparatory phase begins when food or liquid is presented to the oral cavity. Movements of the tongue, lips and teeth form it into a cohesive bolus in preparation for the swallow.

Oral transit phase. The oral transit phase, also called anterior-posterior transit or A-P transit, begins when the tongue transfers the cohesive bolus from the front to the back of the oral cavity. The swallow is initiated by the arrival of the bolus at the back of the tongue.

Pharyngeal phase. When the bolus passes through the faucial pillars (the bilateral arches visible at the back of the mouth), it enters the pharyngeal stage. At this stage multiple structures and muscles become involved. As the bolus reaches the valleculae (folds between the root of the tongue and epiglottis), the epiglottis inverts (epiglottic inversion), covering and protecting the airway. The bolus passes over the epiglottis, through the pyriform sinuses, and through the cricopharyngeus, also commonly referred to as the upper esophageal sphincter (UES), a sphincter muscle of the pharynx and upper esophagus.

Cervical-esophageal stage. The cervical-esophageal phase begins when the bolus enters the esophagus. From there peristaltic muscle contractions carry the material to the stomach for digestion.

Swallowing in Infants

The anatomical and physiological differences between infants and adults affect the swallowing function in several ways:

- The infant's larynx is two or three cervical vertebrae higher than an adult's, which increases the baby's vulnerability to aspiration. The facts that the airway is closer to the oral cavity and that the pharynx is more compact also increase the risk of aspiration.

- The infant's larynx is tucked under the tongue during a swallow, reducing the coordination required to protect the airway. In adults, the larynx is more distal to the tongue base, thus increasing the critical need for integrated movements of several structures for airway protection.

- The uvula and epiglottis are in such close proximity that they make contact, serving two swallowing functions: (a) the contact forms a barrier limiting airflow through the mouth, making infants obligate nasal breathers and allowing them to breathe more continuously during swallowing; and (b) the contact provides a natural protection of the airway while swallowing because the bolus is directed around the lateral edges of the epiglottis and into the pharynx and esophagus.

- Typical nippling in an infant demands a coordinated relationship between sucking, swallowing and breathing. The process of sucking triggers the swallow in such a way that the rate of sucking and the size of the bolus affect the frequency and timing of swallowing. As well, respiration is suppressed during swallowing, which leads to a reduction of respiratory rate and depth of respiration. Infants with atypical breathing patterns may develop atypical sucking patterns to minimize respiratory compromise, and atypical sucking patterns in turn will affect swallowing and breathing patterns.

The evolution of the infant's anatomy into more adult-like anatomy begins around four to six months and continues throughout the first year of life. The larynx descends and the oral cavity opens as the mandible grows, allowing the tongue more room to manipulate a bolus and making possible the transition from liquid to solid consistencies. The separation of the uvula from the epiglottis, along with the descent of the larynx, begins the pathway to epiglottic inversion during swallowing.

Even with a normally functioning system, discoordination or inefficient movement of the structures may cause penetration or aspiration to occur. Aspiration may result from poor bolus control, decreased laryngeal elevation, reduced or absent epiglottic inversion, incomplete vocal cord closure or decreased subglottic pressures. Introduction of a tracheostomy tube places the individual at higher risk for aspiration with swallowing because it tends to restrict laryngeal and epiglottic movement and reduce subglottic pressures.

Influence of a Tracheostomy Tube on Swallowing

Given the very dynamic events that occur with swallowing, even healthy individuals may experience occasional choking or coughing. And, although some individuals with tracheostomy tubes are able to swallow effectively, many patients find swallowing more difficult. An inefficient or ineffective swallow in a tracheostomized patient is most likely due to reductions in subglottic pressure, vocal cord closure or laryngeal sensation, or a combination of all three. The following are common problems caused by the presence of a tracheostomy tube.

Decreased pharyngeal and laryngeal sensation. Tracheostomy tubes tend to decrease pharyngeal sensation due to the reduced or absent airflow into the pharynx. This also reduces stimulation of sensory receptors on the underside of the true vocal cords that contribute to vocal cord closure. This problem is especially acute in the first six months after initial tracheostomy tube placement.

Decreased laryngeal elevation and anterior movement. Tracheostomy tube placement tends to interfere with laryngeal elevation and anterior movement. In most cases the tube "anchors" the trachea to the strap muscles and skin of the neck, restricting elevation of the thyroid cartilage. An inflated tracheal cuff may also "tether" the larynx, impeding laryngeal movement and epiglottic inversion. Ventilator tubing may also interfere with swallowing, because its weight pulls down on the tracheostomy tube, further limiting laryngeal movement. This resistance is difficult to overcome, especially for those who are frail or elderly.

Loss of subglottic pressure. Through its design, the tracheostomy tube creates an open respiratory system. Because of difficulty closing the vocal cords and the escape of exhaled air through the unoccluded tracheostomy tube rather than through the pharynx and larynx as in normal swallows, the increased subglottic pressure necessary for closing the vocal cords to protect against airway penetration cannot be created.

Latent or reduced glottic closure. Reduced laryngeal elevation and sensation, lack of positive subglottic pressure, an inflated tracheal cuff, and reduced vocal cord function all may interfere with vocal cord closure.

Reduced sensory awareness and coordination of respiration with swallowing. Lack of airflow through the pharynx reduces sensation and proprioceptive feedback, meaning that the person is less likely to feel the need to cough. Moreover, individuals who are unable to create elevated subglottic pressure can be expected to have an ineffective or inefficient cough.

Impingement into the esophagus. The inflated tracheal cuff may impinge on the esophagus, especially if it is overinflated (see figure 5.2, page 84). The partial obstruction of the esophagus created by the cuff may slow or impede the peristaltic muscle action that propels the bolus toward the stomach. If sufficiently extreme the constriction may cause a backup of food material that may spill into the airway and potentially be aspirated into the lungs.

Significantly reduced senses of taste and smell. The lack of airflow through the oral and nasal cavities decreases sensations of smell and taste, which may reduce an individual's appetite and ultimately affect nutritional status.

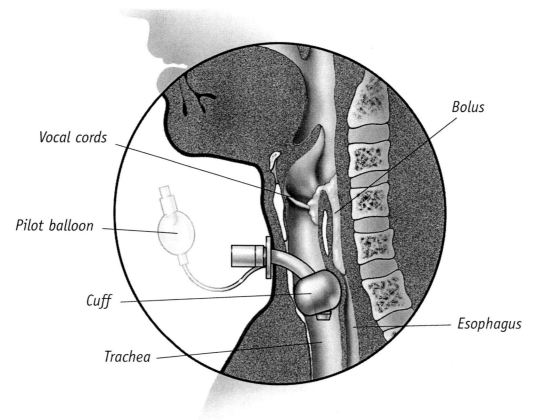

Vocal cords

Pilot balloon

Cuff

Trachea

Bolus

Esophagus

Figure 5.2. Overinflated cuff pressing into the esophagus and obstructing the passage of a bolus.

It is crucial to remember the fundamental differences between tracheostomy and endotracheal (ET) tubes. Due to the nature of endotracheal intubation, swallowing is not an option for individuals with these types of tubes. Because the vocal cords are held open by the tube, all protection of the airway is lost. The ET tube also obstructs the oral cavity and requires an inflated cuff to be effective for ventilation.

Issues Surrounding the Tracheostomy Cuff

As mentioned previously, the cuff of a tracheostomy tube can be problematic during swallowing. It transfers the weight of the tracheostomy tube to the trachea, potentially anchoring the thyroid cartilage and restricting full elevation of the larynx. As well, the continual friction between the inflated cuff and the tracheal tissue during swallowing may lead to necrosis (tissue death) on the tracheal wall as well as the development of tracheoesophageal fistulas (see figure 5.3). As described previously, overinflation of the tracheostomy tube cuff may force the posterior wall of the trachea backward into the esophagus, creating an obstruction (as shown in figure 5.2). On the other hand, the folds of an underinflated or deflated cuff create a site for poten-

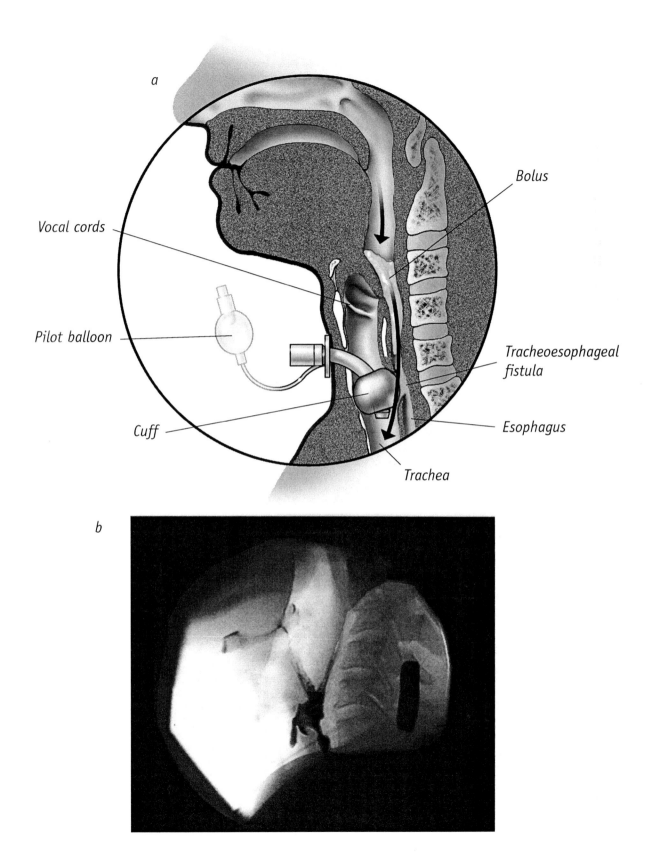

a

Bolus

Vocal cords

Pilot balloon

Tracheoesophageal fistula

Cuff

Esophagus

Trachea

b

Figure 5.3. Tracheoesophageal fistula: (a) illustration showing potential for aspiration directly from the esophagus; (b) fistula observed during a modified barium swallow.

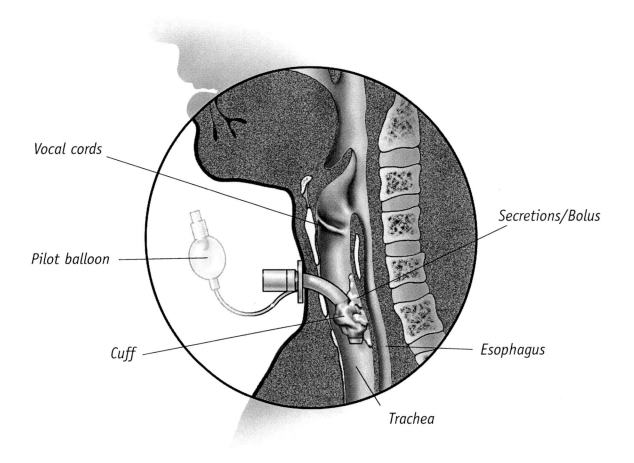

Vocal cords

Secretions/Bolus

Pilot balloon

Cuff

Esophagus

Trachea

Figure 5.4. Aspirated material pooling in and around an underinflated tracheostomy cuff.

tial pooling of material or saliva, increasing the risk of delayed aspiration (see figure 5.4, page 86).

There is a major misconception concerning the role of a tracheostomy cuff in protecting the airway from aspiration. Many medical professionals consider an inflated tracheostomy cuff a foolproof means of protection from aspirated material. By definition, however, aspiration is "the entry of foreign material into the airway, past the level of the vocal folds" (Dikeman and Kazandjian 1995, p. 335). Since the tracheostomy tube and cuff are below the level of the true vocal cords, any material that reaches the cuff has *already been aspirated*. Therefore, the cuff has not protected the airway, although it may postpone or slow the fall of material so it can be suctioned out before reaching the lungs. Even under the best of circumstances, there is still potential for material to leak past the inflated cuff and make its way into the lungs. It is important that you, as a speech-language pathologist, educate the interdisciplinary team about laryngeal anatomy and emphasize that any material passing below the level of the true vocal cords constitutes aspiration and is potentially dangerous.

Swallowing Assessment with a Tracheostomy Tube

Certain considerations will determine whether the time is appropriate for a swallowing evaluation. The following information can be obtained through a thorough medical chart review, consultation with the physician and respiratory therapists, and interviews with the patient and family.

Is the patient able to participate in a swallowing evaluation? How alert is he or she? Will the patient be able to follow commands? To sit upright? As with any swallowing evaluation, it is important that the patient be awake and able to participate in the evaluation. Positioning is particularly important with patients who are tracheostomized. The individual may not be able to sit at a ninety-degree angle, but ideally he or she should be positioned as close to this angle as possible. Sometimes it is necessary for the evaluation to be performed under the patient's "typical" circumstances or at the angle of the patient's preference. For example, a patient may have a restriction that the height of the head of the bed is not to exceed forty-five degrees.

Is the patient able to tolerate cuff deflation and a speaking valve? Recall that repeated swallowing with an inflated cuff could lead to the development of a tracheoesophageal fistula. If a patient is able to tolerate a speaking valve, the valve may improve swallowing ability, as discussed previously. Therefore, before initiating swallowing trials, the first priority is to increase cuff deflation tolerance and speaking valve use.

Modified Evan's Blue Dye Test

The **modified Evan's blue dye test** was developed as an indicator of whether a patient with a tracheostomy tube is aspirating tube feedings. Although there is very little research regarding the modified Evan's blue dye test, most facilities with a large tracheostomy/ventilator population are familiar with this protocol and include it in their repertoire of assessments.

The word "modified" in the name refers to dyeing liquids, purees, and solids with blue (or green) food coloring, feeding the dyed material to the patient, and subsequently suctioning the trachea. Blue or green dye is used because it is easily detected and cannot be mistaken for other bodily fluids (mucus, blood). Traditionally methylene blue has been used, but because some patients have an allergic reaction to it, the use of household food coloring is becoming more common. A second variation that is becoming popular is to use foods or liquids that have naturally distinctive colors (such as chocolate pudding, blueberry yogurt, or grape juice). This option is used most in facilities that discourage the overuse of food coloring. Secretions in the suction tubing (and around the tracheostoma) are examined for traces of blue. Any change in the color of the secretions (even traces of pale blue) is a sign of aspirated material. Secretions from later suctionings should also be monitored for blue coloring, because material may temporarily pool at any of several sites for a time before being aspirated. A complete protocol for modified Evan's blue dye test follows in the next section.

A variation of this test is to place blue or green food coloring directly on the patient's tongue. If suctioned secretions from the trachea or around the tracheostoma are color-tinged (either immediately or up to several hours later), this is a good indication that the patient is aspirating his or her own secretions. This is important information; if a patient is unable to swallow his or her oral secretions safely, then oral nutrition is not appropriate at this time.

An advantage of the modified Evan's blue dye test is that it is noninvasive and very inexpensive to perform. A disadvantage is that it is not 100 percent reliable: a patient may have a negative blue-dye test (no blue-tinged secretions) and still be aspirating (false negative result). Because of the potential health risks of aspiration, if a patient passes the blue-dye test, it is preferable to conduct an instrumental assessment (such as a modified barium swallow) to confirm the lack of aspiration. If no formal assessment procedures are available, we recommend a protocol in which a patient must pass three blue-dye tests with each consistency prior to the initiation of oral nutrition. Because of the potential for a patient's condition to fluctuate, trials preferably should be scheduled on different days and at various times of day.

Protocol for Modified Evan's Blue Dye Test

1. Obtain authorization from the patient's physician to perform the blue-dye test, documenting that it will assist in identifying whether the patient is at risk for aspirating oral secretions or oral nutrition.

2. Coordinate the testing schedule with a respiratory therapist or nurse, who will suction the patient. If patient is ventilator-dependent, a respiratory therapist must be present to deflate the tracheostomy tube cuff for suctioning and to monitor ventilator settings and alarms (see chapter 6 for further discussion).

3. If the patient is currently NPO (receiving nothing by mouth) and the aspiration of secretions is a potential concern, place two or three drops (about 0.2–0.4 cc) of blue food coloring on the patient's tongue.

4. If the patient is cleared for trials of oral food or liquid, place two or three drops of blue food coloring in food or liquid. Determine the consistency and amount of food or liquid to present based on the individual's status and personal goals. It is important to present a sufficient amount of material to reveal aspiration if present. (For example, one ice chip is not sufficient to reveal aspiration.)

5. Have the nurse or respiratory therapist suction the trachea immediately after presentation of the food or liquid, again two or three minutes later, ten minutes later, and finally thirty minutes later.

6. Inspect any secretions expectorated from the tracheostomy tube, suctioned from the airway, or leaking from the tracheostoma. If any blue is noted, document this on the tracking sheet (see page 90), which should be kept bedside.

7. If no blue-tinged secretions are suctioned or expectorated, continue with swallowing trials, presenting a variety of consistencies if appropriate and suctioning immediately following each presentation. Bear in mind that if you present several different consistencies during the same trial, it may be difficult to determine which consistency was aspirated. One solution may be to use different colors for different consistencies (for example, undyed chocolate pudding and blue-dyed water).

8. Based on the results of this and subsequent testing sessions, make recommendations regarding the patient's potential for oral nutrition and any limitations in consistency, texture or amount.

Cautions

- Notify the nursing and respiratory staff whenever you perform a modified Evan's blue dye test because the bluish tinge to the lips could be confused with hypoxia (not getting enough oxygen) and the medical staff may begin unnecessary efforts to ventilate the person. Request that nursing and respiratory staff continue to monitor the suctioned material for signs of dye and document any unusual findings.

- In some facilities, nutrition delivered via tube feedings may be dyed with blue food coloring. If so choose another color of dye so as to distinguish whether aspirated material, if any, resulted from the oral trials or the tube feedings.

- Although good oral hygiene is especially important with patients who are tracheostomized to decrease the risk of infection, it is important to suspend cleaning of the oral cavity, specifically the tongue, while the patient is undergoing a modified Evan's blue dye test on secretions. The cleaning will remove the dye, negating the test.

Blue Dye Swallowing Assessment Tracking

Patient's name:		Date:
Patient's ID:		
Consistency tested:		Color:

Instructions: [ ] Deflate cuff   [ ] Leave cuff inflated   [ ] Cuffless

[ ] Suction every _____ hours

[ ] Beginning date/time:

[ ] Ending date/time:

Date/Time	Aspiration Noted (+ or -)	Amount	Comments	Initials

Speech-language pathologist:

Tracheostomy Tubes and Ventilator Dependence in Adults and Children—VanDahm and Sparks-Walsh

© 2002 by PRO-ED, Inc.

Glucose Strip Testing for Aspiration

Another noninvasive procedure for identifying aspiration in patients who are tracheostomized is the use of glucose strips (see figure 5.5). The essence of the evaluation is to obtain a baseline measure of the glucose content in the patient's secretions, then compare it to the glucose content in secretions obtained after the patient has swallowed a sugar-laden bolus. Again, no research has been published on the efficacy of this procedure with oral intake of food. There is, however, one article discussing the use of glucose strip testing to monitor aspiration with tube feedings (Kinsey et al. 1994).

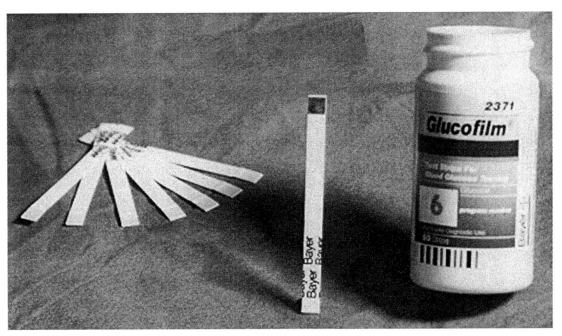

Figure 5.5. Glucofilm® Test Strips for glucose testing. (Courtesy of Bayer, Inc.)

Protocol for Use of Glucose Strips

Materials needed: gloves, cotton swabs, glucose strips, sugar-laden food or liquid

1. Remove the inner cannula from the tracheostomy tube. (Note: If the patient is on a ventilator, make sure you are trained by either the respiratory therapist or nursing staff. Removal of the inner cannula will temporarily reduce ventilation to the patient. Complete steps 1 and 2 before any serious complications result.)

2. Using a swab, swipe secretions from inside the tube and place on a glucose strip, then immediately replace the inner cannula. This will provide you with the baseline glucose content of the patient's secretions.

3. Allow the patient to drink a sugar-laden liquid (such as regular soda), eat a sweetened food or suck on a piece of sugared candy (preferably a Lifesaver® or

other candy with a hole so you can attach a length of dental floss to prevent accidental ingestion).

4. Wait several minutes, then repeat steps 1 and 2 with a fresh glucose strip.

5. Examine the two strips for any variation in color between them. If any change is noted, this is an indication of aspiration.

6. If no signs of aspiration are noted, repeat steps 1 and 2 up to ten minutes later, depending on the consistency of food or liquid presented. Confirming the results with other evaluation methods is recommended before clearing the patient for oral nutrition.

Cervical Auscultation

Cervical auscultation is another noninvasive method of evaluating the swallowing mechanism. The trained clinician places a stethoscope on the patient's larynx during the swallow. With sufficient training, the presence or absence of a swallow may be detected, as well as breath sounds that indicate a patient has a compromised airway. This procedure could be incorporated into the bedside swallowing evaluation. Some clinicians use it along with the modified Evan's blue dye test, especially for patients who cannot undergo a modified barium swallow (MBS) study or fiberoptic endoscopic evaluation of swallowing (FEES®).

Videofluoroscopy

Most speech-language pathologists consider the modified barium swallow (MBS) study, also known as a videofluorographic swallow study (VFSS), the gold standard for evaluating dysphagia. It is the most widely used and generally accepted procedure for assessing swallowing. The MBS is performed in a radiology suite, typically with a radiologist present. The speech-language pathologist may or may not be involved, depending on the setting. Some facilities allow a great deal of involvement while others permit the speech-language pathologist to observe and offer recommendations only. Typically all different food textures are evaluated (thin and thick liquids, puree, solids and pills) because an individual may be able to swallow certain consistencies safely but not others. Positioning and compensatory strategies may be assessed for their effectiveness in improving swallowing function. Suctioning equipment should be on hand for immediate suctioning of any material aspirated during this study. Especially with individuals who are ventilator-dependent, we recommend that a respiratory therapist or nurse be available for respiratory management during and after the procedure.

An MBS is particularly useful in identifying silent aspiration, determining the cause of aspiration, and developing swallowing strategies that reduce or eliminate aspiration potential. For patients who can tolerate a speaking valve, the valve should be in place during the study to provide optimal conditions. For all patients it is preferable to deflate the tracheostomy cuff for the study, because of its potential to interfere with swallowing. (The cuff must, of course, be deflated if a speaking valve is being used.)

The advantage of an MBS is that it provides a picture of the complete swallowing mechanism. Most oral and pharyngeal structures are visible, and the study can be videotaped for review and discussion with the patient, family and other medical professionals on the team. Disadvantages are the expense of the procedure, the radiation exposure to the patient and clinician, and the fact that it is a time-limited examination (meaning that fatigue-related swallowing issues will not be apparent in the short time of the study).

▉ Fiberoptic Endoscopic Evaluation of Swallowing (FEES®)

This fiberoptic evaluation procedure involves passing a flexible endoscope (see figure 5.6) through the nares into the pharynx above the epiglottis. From this position, the patient's swallow can be observed from above. The various food textures are dyed with green or blue food coloring so they can be distinguished from bodily tissues and fluid. One advantage of FEES® is that the evaluation can continue as long as necessary without exposing the patient to radiation. Whereas the MBS evaluation is brief due to radiation exposure, FEES® can be used to evaluate patients for fatigue by leaving the endoscope in place during an entire meal. FEES® can also be conducted at the patient's bedside. One disadvantage of FEES® is the inability to observe exactly why or when during the swallow a patient aspirates, or to quantify the amount of material aspirated.

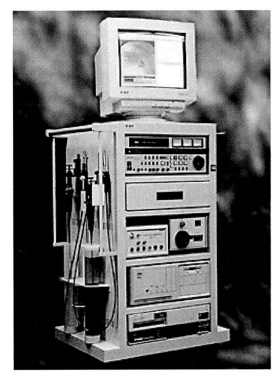

Figure 5.6. Swallowing workstation used for FEES®. (Courtesy of Kay Elemetrics Corp.)

Strategies to Increase Swallowing Safety and Efficiency with a Tracheostomy Tube

Several different strategies can facilitate safe and efficient swallowing for someone who has a tracheostomy tube. (Additional strategies for patients on a ventilator will be addressed in chapter 6.) Each patient's current medical status dictates which options are viable in that particular case. Decisions regarding these strategies should be made in consultation with the patient and the interdisciplinary team.

Cuff Deflation

Cuff deflation is an important step in improving the safety and efficiency of swallowing in any patient who is tracheostomized. As mentioned earlier, tracheoesophageal fistulas may develop through long-term friction between the cuff and tracheal wall, thus creating another route for aspiration (see figure 5.3, page 85). Deflating the cuff allows the tracheostomy tube to move more freely within the trachea, facilitating adequate elevation of the larynx. Because patients vary in how well they tolerate having the cuff deflated, systematic cuff-deflation trials should be conducted. A typical trial begins with cuff deflation for one minute and continues for gradually longer time periods while the patient is monitored for behavioral signs of distress (see page 71). Trials can continue as long as the patient tolerates them or as indicated by the physician.

Speaking Valves

We recommend that whenever possible the patient should be able to tolerate at least one hour of Passy-Muir Speaking Valve (PMV) use before swallowing therapy is initiated. Because of the "no-leak" design of these valves, they normalize pressure in the pharynx by closing the airway during exhalation. This helps normalize swallowing physiology, which may improve the swallowing process and decrease the risk for aspiration. This benefit is documented exclusively with Passy-Muir Tracheostomy Speaking Valves, not with other "open position" one-way speaking valves (Dettelbach et al. 1995).

Mendelsohn Maneuver

The Mendelsohn maneuver is used for individuals with reduced laryngeal elevation, a common problem in tracheostomy. Reduced laryngeal elevation often causes residue to collect in the pharynx as well as reducing epiglottic inversion (decreasing protection of the airway); using this maneuver may help clear this residue and promote epiglottic movement. The strategy requires the patient to swallow, then consciously keep the larynx in its elevated position while swallowing a second time, before relaxing and allowing the larynx to drop. The Mendelsohn maneuver can be difficult to perform, and typically only patients who are cognitively alert will grasp the concept and be able to perform it successfully. Moreover, due to the amount of effort required for each swallow, patients may fatigue quickly when using this strategy. This strategy may also be ineffective for patients who have decreased pharyngeal sensation (a typical side effect of a tracheostomy tube) and who are unable to sense premature spillage.

■ Removal of the Tracheostomy Tube

It seems intuitive that, if a patient was swallowing normally prior to placement of a tracheostomy tube, removal of the tube would allow normal swallowing once again. Unfortunately, this is not always the case. Incidents leading up to the placement of the tracheostomy tube and the course of the patient medical condition may make swallowing difficult even after the tube is removed, although removal of the tube may remove a structural barrier that had been contributing to the patient's dysphagia. The patient should be warned that there are no guarantees, so that he or she will be prepared if swallowing function still is impaired after decannulation (removal of the tracheostomy tube). Similarly, individuals who have been eating by mouth with the tracheostomy tube in place may experience temporary dysphagia when the tube is removed due to the open stoma. It is recommended that all oral nutrition and hydration be withheld, if possible, until the stoma has closed and no air leakage is heard or felt through the stoma during speech. Every person heals at a different rate, but this typically requires about twenty-four hours.

Removal of the tracheostomy tube is a medical decision made by the physician. It is certainly within our scope of practice as speech-language pathologists to report that removal of tracheostomy tube may normalize swallowing. Reasons for keeping the tracheostomy tube in place may take precedence over eating orally, however. It is important to remember that even though taking nutrition orally may be a high priority for the patient or family, doing so may not be in the patient's best interest. Other medical issues, such as resolving aspiration pneumonia or allowing healing after a surgery, may take precedence. Careful and thorough patient and family education may be necessary to give them a realistic understanding of the patient's current level of function, the risks and potential complications of reinitiating oral feeding too early, and quality-of-life issues.

Conclusion

Dysphagia can be a precarious disorder, and the risks and complications are increased when a tracheostomy tube is present. Decreased laryngeal elevation, reduced pharyngeal sensation, and the change in subglottic pressures must all be recognized as potential pitfalls when evaluating the swallowing function of a patient who is tracheotomized. Careful assessment with clinical bedside evaluations and instrumental evaluations, well-thought-out recommendations and the targeted use of strategies to enhance swallowing can be very instrumental in assisting the patient to eat safely and efficiently while tracheostomized.

Chapter 6
Mechanical Ventilation

Although it is not within a speech-language pathologist's scope of practice to set up and maintain a ventilator, it is beneficial to have a basic understanding of ventilator modes and settings, what the alarms mean, and how a ventilator may affect communication and swallowing in a patient with complex medical needs. This chapter provides the foundation for clinicians to understand ventilators and use that information in therapeutic planning and intervention. It is also wise to cultivate a rapport with the professionals specializing in ventilator management—namely, pulmonologists, respiratory therapists and specially trained nursing staff—who can assist with problem solving and evaluating the patient's potential for treatment.

How a Ventilator Works

By definition, mechanical ventilation is the movement of air into and out of the lungs through artificial means. Although mechanical ventilation does not address the underlying medical issue that prevents the patient from breathing independently, it does support gas exchange until the medical issue can be resolved or stabilized. For example, ventilator support may be needed for a person who has sustained a significant stroke and has gone into respiratory failure. The ventilator will support respiratory function, but will not cure the stroke that caused the respiratory failure to occur.

As you will recall from chapter 1, the process of breathing involves inhalation, an active expansion of the chest that pulls air into the lungs, and exhalation, a passive recoil that pushes air out of the lungs. There are patients, however, who have difficulty exhaling due to poor elastic recoil of the alveoli. For example, damage from smoking can cause the alveoli to lose their elasticity. Inability to adequately empty the lungs of spent air, which contains a higher concentration of carbon dioxide, results in a buildup of carbon dioxide in the bloodstream. These patients may need long-term ventilator support to compensate for their difficulty in exhaling.

Types of Ventilators

There are two types of ventilators: negative-pressure and positive-pressure ventilators. Both operate by creating inhalation and allowing the natural elasticity of the alveoli to move the air out of the lungs. Negative-pressure ventilators (for example, the old "iron lung") move air into the lungs by creating negative pressure around the chest. The resulting vacuum causes a rush of air into the lungs in order to equalize the negative pressure. The positive-pressure ventilators most commonly used today simply force air into the lungs. This forcing of air, if not properly measured and regularly monitored, may lead to complications such as trauma to the alveoli (termed barotraumas) or pressure on the vessels surrounding the heart, creating a reduction in cardiac output. Therefore, an individual on a ventilator must be closely followed.

Movement of air into and out of the lungs is typically, though not always, accomplished through an artificial airway. Exceptions are cases where the person requires a ventilator only at night (for example, due to sleep apnea), when the necessary ventilation is given via a special facemask or nasal system instead of an endotracheal or tracheostomy tube. (This system will be discussed further under "Bilevel Continuous Positive Airway Pressure" on page 101.) The ventilator is connected to the artificial airway via flexible tubing. The connection between the tubing and the artificial airway varies depending on the brand of equipment and the standard practice of the particular facility. If the patient needs to be suctioned frequently, an in-line or closed suctioning unit is used (in which the suctioning catheter remains sterile for up to forty-eight hours). This unit allows suctioning without disconnecting the patient from the ventilator. The ventilator tubing is attached to the suctioning unit as shown in figure 6.1. Tubing can also be attached to the airway tube with a flexible tubing adapter. A commonly used brand is an Omni-Flex (see figure 6.2). This small adapter allows the patient some movement without pulling against the airway tube.

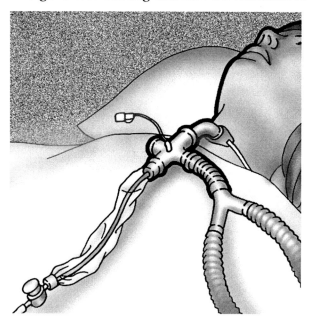

Figure 6.1. In-line suctioning unit.

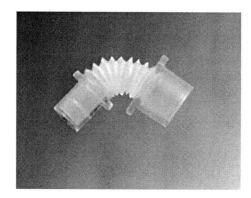

Figure 6.2. Omni-Flex connector. (Courtesy of Allegiance Healthcare)

Another differentiating feature of ventilators is portability. Many ventilators used in a hospital are not considered portable and have little if any battery backup. Ventilators such as the PB 7200, Bear and Infant Star are common brands of nonportable systems. Portable ventilators such as the LP 6 and LP 10, as well as the new Lap Top Ventilator (LTV) 950 and 1000 models, are typically used for patients who are at

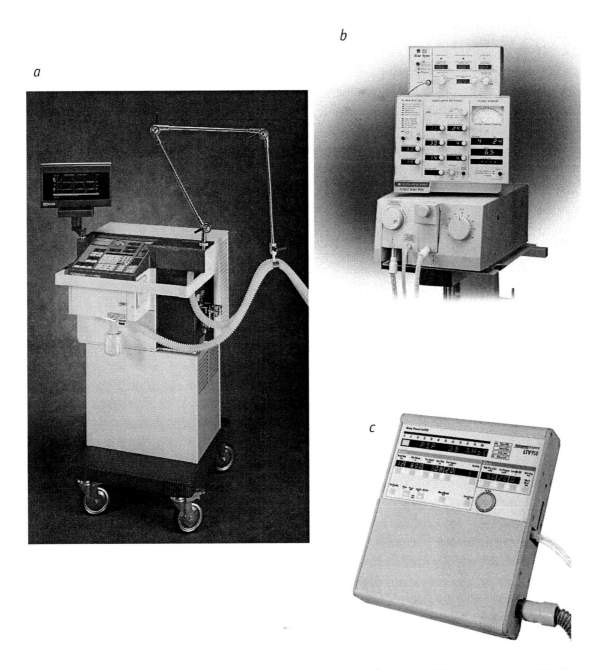

Figure 6.3. Common brands of ventilators: (a) PB 7200 (Reprinted by permission of Nellcor Puritan Bennett, Pleasanton, CA); (b) Infant Star (Reprinted by permission of Nellcor Puritan Bennett, Inc., Pleasanton, CA); (c) LTV 950 (Courtesy of Pulmonetic Systems, Inc.)

home and need to be mobile in order to go to school or doctor's appointments or accomplish activities of daily living. These portable systems are smaller (in fact, the new LTV 1000 can be hoisted over the shoulder), can be mounted onto a special tray on the back of a wheelchair or stowed under a stroller, and have a backup battery that can last for a couple of hours if needed (see figure 6.3, page 99). When someone on a ventilator is discharged from the hospital, the patient and family members should be advised to notify their local utility companies and fire and police stations of the presence of a ventilator in the home. This will put them on a priority list for power restoration and emergency services.

Most current ventilators have a display showing the mode, rate and volume at which the unit is set (these terms will be defined below). Some ventilators also show data about spontaneous breaths the patient is attempting. It is important to familiarize yourself with the displays and control panels of different ventilators so if a ventilator alarm sounds while you are providing therapy to a patient, you can quickly determine the reason (see figure 6.3, page 99).

Ventilator Parameters and Terminology

Rate. Rate refers to the number of breaths delivered to the patient by the ventilator per minute. It is measured in bpm, for breaths per minute. Recall that the normal respiratory rate for adults is twelve to twenty bpm; for children it is thirty to forty bpm and for infants sixty to eighty bpm. An individual's ventilatory rate is set within these parameters, allowing for any spontaneous breaths. As the individual weans from ventilatory support and is able to breathe more effectively on his or her own, the rate is reduced. The rate is usually written as a number next to the specified ventilation mode on the physician's order or prescription. (For example, SIMV 12 means synchronized intermittent mechanical ventilation mode with a rate of twelve breaths per minute; PS 8 means pressure support mode with a rate of eight breaths per minute.)

Tidal volume. Tidal volume (abbreviated TV or V_t), is the amount of air moved into and out of the respiratory tract during a breathing cycle. The amount prescribed is based on a guideline of ten to fifteen milliliters per kilogram of body weight. For example, an individual weighing 70 kg would typically have a tidal volume of 700–1,050 ml. The ventilator measures how much air is being delivered to the individual as well as how much air is returned to the ventilator. These two measures should remain very similar. If the measures diverge, the ventilator alarm will sound (typically the low tidal volume, low exhaled volume, or apnea alarms will be triggered).

Positive end-expiratory pressure (PEEP). PEEP is a minimum pressure that is maintained within the alveoli to prevent them from collapsing at the end of every breath (thus the name "end-expiratory pressure"). PEEP is usually indicated with mechanical ventilation because tracheal intubation holds the larynx constantly open and can lead to alveolar collapse, termed atelectasis, unless supplementary pressure is provided. Atelectasis decreases lung elasticity and inhibits oxygenation. Therapeutic uses of PEEP help to prevent and sometimes reverse atelectasis. Normal ranges of PEEP are between 2 and 5 cm H_2O. As discussed in chapter 4, the Passy-Muir Speaking Valve (PMV) claims to maintain a physiologic PEEP of 5 cm H_2O, making the provision of PEEP unnecessary while the patient is using PMV in-line with the ventilator unless the desired PEEP is greater than 5 cm H_2O (Passy et al. 1993).

Peak inspiratory pressure (PIP). Peak inspiratory pressure is the highest level of pressure the individual achieves during inspiration, measured in cm H_2O. The peak pressure is different for every breath; for example, coughing causes the PIP to increase. Some individuals, particularly infants, require a set PIP limit to prevent barotrauma and damage to the lungs.

Fraction of inspired oxygen (FiO_2). FiO_2 measures the percentage of oxygen in the gas being provided by the ventilator. Recall from chapter 2 that typical environmental air, or room air, is 21 percent oxygen. A patient may receive anywhere from 21 percent to 100 percent FiO_2, depending on how much is required to maintain adequate oxygenation. However, recall from chapter 4 that anyone who requires more than 40 percent FiO_2 (or 40 percent O_2 while not on the ventilator), may not be a good candidate for intensive therapy using a speaking valve until the need for supplementary oxygen can be reduced.

Inspiratory-to-expiratory ratio (I:E ratio). I:E ratio is the ratio of the length of inspiration to the length of expiration. Typically the I:E ratio programmed into the ventilator is patterned after the normal spontaneous ratio of 1:2 (one second for inspiration and two seconds for expiration). This ratio may be changed if needed. For example, patients with chronic obstructive pulmonary disease (COPD) may require a longer expiratory time of 1:3 or 1:4, and infants have a shorter inspiratory time of .3 to .7 seconds.

Sensitivity. Sensitivity refers to the amount of effort the patient must exhibit to initiate a spontaneous breath, measured by the amount of negative pressure created within the respiratory tract. The typical sensitivity value is -2 cm H_2O.

Bilevel continuous positive airway pressure (BiPAP). BiPAP is a short-term, noninvasive procedure used to improve oxygenation when the patient is capable of spontaneous ventilation. If it is unsuccessful in improving oxygenation, intubation and ventilation are initiated. Rather than being delivered through a ventilator, BiPAP can be given through nasal pillows (similar to nasal prongs but the tubing goes up over the top of the head rather than around the ears), through a specialized nasal mask or through a mask that covers both the mouth and the nose. Again, BiPAP is used when oxygenation is the concern rather than ventilation. BiPAP uses inspiratory and expiratory pressures and is set up as a rate. This rate is written as a fraction of inspiratory pressure over expiratory pressure (with inspiratory pressure usually being greater than expiratory pressure). BiPAP is defined here because you may see the term in patients' charts and because it is often confused with CPAP, which is a mode of ventilation defined below. It is important to remember that BiPAP is not used in conjunction with a ventilator.

Weaning. Weaning is a process of systematically reducing ventilator settings and modes to decrease the support provided by the ventilator while increasing the respiratory work performed by the patient in preparation for removing the patient from the ventilator. One study has indicated that weaning success may be improved through the use of the Passy-Muir Speaking Valve (Frey and Wood 1991).

Modes of Mechanical Ventilation

There are two basic modes of ventilation. In full ventilatory support mode, the ventilator carries out all the work of breathing. In spontaneous, or partial, ventilatory support mode, the patient shares the work of breathing with the ventilator. With a range of possible combinations between full ventilatory support and no ventilatory support, there are five commonly prescribed modes, which are described below and summarized in table 6.1 (page 106). The physician selects the most appropriate mode and parameters for a patient based on how much of the work of breathing the individual should or can maintain. In making this decision, the physician must consider such factors as the volume of air the patient should be taking into the lungs, how much pressure the alveoli can handle based on their elasticity, how much spontaneous breathing the patient can do and how much supplemental oxygen is needed to maintain an adequate oxygen saturation level in the blood. By monitoring the data on the ventilator control panels, obtaining arterial blood gas draws (ABGs) from the patient, and observing the patient's physical symptoms, the physician can determine whether the individual's respiratory needs are being met and adjust the ventilator modes and parameters accordingly. The following are the most commonly prescribed modes, which are used with the parameters just described.

Controlled Mechanical Ventilation (CMV)

CMV is the full ventilator support mode, in which the ventilator performs all the work of breathing. The ventilator is set according to the physician's orders to deliver a fixed tidal volume and respiratory rate, regardless of whether the patient attempts any spontaneous breaths. CMV is used for patients who exhibit little or no respiratory effort or are incapable of initiating spontaneous breaths due to the complexity of their medical condition. Controlled mechanical ventilation is typically used with patients who are comatose, are in the initial stages of a serious trauma, have a high-level spinal cord injury or have an end-stage pulmonary or degenerative disease. Sometimes patients are placed on this mode when chemical sedation is necessary and neuromuscular blocking agents are used; for example, during surgery or if the patient is resisting medical intervention.

Advantage: The ventilator performs all the work of breathing for those patients who are unable to maintain their own respiratory support.

Disadvantages: Long-term use of this mode may lead to muscle atrophy or weakening, since the ventilator does all the work of breathing. The ventilator does not compensate for any spontaneous breaths the patient takes. When the patient initiates a breath that is followed by the preset tidal volume being delivered by the ventilator, this phenomenon is termed breath stacking. The extra air forced into the lungs in breath stacking may lead to hyperventilation of the lungs, barotraumas, or excessive pressure on the heart and blood vessels.

Assist-Controlled Ventilation (AC)

AC is a controlled ventilatory support mode. Again, a preset volume and respiratory rate are maintained regardless of the patient's spontaneous efforts. Should the patient initiate a breath, however, the ventilator will complete that breath with the full preset volume. In this mode, the patient may have two respiratory rates: a spontaneous rate and a mechanical rate. For example, if the ventilator is set at a rate of fifteen breaths per minute (bpm) the ventilator will provide all fifteen breaths. Should the patient initiate three spontaneous breaths, the ventilator will supplement those spontaneous breaths to reach the prescribed tidal volume and also provide the set rate of fifteen breaths. The AC mode of ventilation is typically used with patients who are able to initiate breathing but may not have the ability to take in a full breath. Patients with muscle fatigue are also good candidates for this mode of ventilation.

Advantages: AC can be used with very sick patients who are unable to tolerate much of the work of breathing. The ventilator will automatically provide the preset respiratory rate should the patient stop breathing or breathe too slowly.

Disadvantages: This mode tends to create higher positive pressure in the thorax than other modes do. It also can lead to muscle deterioration if the patient is unable to provide any spontaneous breaths.

Synchronized Intermittent Mandatory Ventilation (SIMV)

SIMV also uses a preset volume and rate but is considered a spontaneous mode of ventilation. The difference is that the ventilator is programmed to recognize spontaneous breaths and incorporate them into or synchronize them with the preset rate without hyperventilation. The set tidal volume is delivered only on breaths initiated by the ventilator, not those initiated by the patient. Thus if the patient breathes spontaneously, the number of mechanical breaths delivered by the ventilator per minute is reduced accordingly.

Advantages: This mode eliminates breath stacking and lowers intrathoracic pressures. It also supports muscle retraining and strengthening, which is necessary for weaning from the ventilator.

Disadvantages: SIMV may increase the work of breathing since the preset volume is delivered only on mechanical breaths. If the patient's breaths are shallow, he or she must breathe more often.

Pressure Support Ventilation (PS)

PS is a spontaneous mode of ventilation that does not provide any preset breath rate or tidal volume. Instead, this mode assists the patient's spontaneous breaths with a preset amount of pressure during the inspiratory phase of breathing. The tidal volume inhaled may differ from breath to breath because this is dependent on the patient not on the ventilator. However, the added pressure support will enable the patient to take a deeper breath (larger volume) than would be possible independently. This mode would commonly be used for a patient who is able to initiate an adequate number of breaths but is unable to inflate the lungs adequately. This mode allows the patient to initiate the breath but provides extra pressure to increase the tidal volume of the breath. This mode can be used alone or in combination with the SIMV or CPAP/PEEP modes (to be discussed later). If PS is used alone, the patient must have an adequate rate of spontaneous breathing attempts because there is no preset rate or volume of air to be delivered should the patient fail to initiate an adequate number of breaths.

Advantages: PS decreases the work of breathing but allows the patient to build respiratory muscle strength, making it a good tool in weaning from a ventilator. This mode can be used alone or with other modes of ventilation.

Disadvantage: If used alone, PS provides no established volume or rate if the patient's breathing should slow or stop.

Continuous Positive Airway Pressure (CPAP)

CPAP is considered a spontaneous mode of ventilation that provides a specific rate and tidal volume. It is used to prevent alveolar collapse, thus allowing for more efficient gas exchange and better oxygenation. It provides a set amount of positive pressure during both the inhalation and exhalation cycles of spontaneous breaths, which prevents the alveoli from completely deflating between breaths. A patient who can take in an adequate tidal volume but is unable to maintain oxygenation is a good candidate for this mode.

Advantages: CPAP prevents collapse of the airway or alveoli and enhances oxygenation. It is often used during the weaning process.

Disadvantages: It provides no preset volume or rate of breathing as a backup should the patient's breathing slow or stop.

Pressure Control (PC)

PC is a mode of ventilation used to overcome the resistance to airflow caused by the tracheostomy tube and the length of tubing connecting it to the ventilator. By taking a spontaneous breath, the patient triggers the ventilator to deliver a preset amount of pressure, which is designed to achieve a desired tidal volume. This mode is often used with infants to reduce the work of breathing and can be used in combination with other modes of ventilation (with the exception of pressure support).

Advantages: The ventilator will automatically return to the preset respiratory rate should the patient stop breathing. PC mode helps to limit the positive pressure in the thorax. It reduces or eliminates the work of breathing.

Disadvantages: This mode controls the amount of pressure provided but not the tidal volume or rate, so it does not guarantee that the patient will receive a desired tidal volume or specific number of breaths per minute. PC cannot be used in combination with pressure support.

Ventilator Alarms

The function of a ventilator alarm is to alert the caregiver of a change in ventilatory status. Although the alarms vary depending on the brand of ventilator, it is very important to be able to identify the reason why an alarm has triggered and to know what actions to take to remedy the problem. It is also important that family members be taught the different alarms so that they can alert the appropriate professionals if necessary.

Table 6.1. Comparison chart of modes of ventilation

Ventilation type	Controlled Mechanical (CMV)	Assist-Controlled (AC)	Synchronized Intermittent Mandatory (SIMV)	Pressure Support (PS)	Pressure Control (PC)
	Controlled	Controlled	Spontaneous	Spontaneous	Controlled
Tidal volume delivered (assuming physician order of Vt 800 ml)	Fixed volume of 800 ml delivered for all ventilator breaths regardless of spontaneous breaths (if any)	Fixed volume of 800 ml delivered for all ventilator breaths; spontaneous breaths augmented to 800 ml	Fixed volume of 800 ml delivered for ventilator breaths only; spontaneous breaths are whatever volume the patient can achieve independently	No fixed tidal volume; Vt differs with each spontaneous breath; ventilator provides a specified amount of pressure during inspiration	No fixed tidal volume
Respiratory rate (assuming physician order of 10 bpm)	Fixed rate of 10 bpm delivered by ventilator regardless of patient's spontaneous breaths (if any)	Fixed rate of 10 bpm delivered by ventilator regardless of spontaneous breaths (if any)	Ventilator incorporates any spontaneous breaths to maintain a fixed rate of 10 (For example, if patient takes 3 spontaneous breaths, the ventilator will give 7 breaths.)	No fixed rate delivered by ventilator; patient initiates all breaths; often used in combination with CPAP or SIMV modes	No fixed rate; often used in combination with other modes (except PS) in which respiratory rate is specified.

Important Guidelines for Ventilator Alarms

Do not reset an alarm without identifying the cause. In some settings, it may be wisest to allow the alarm to continue to sound so that the appropriate healthcare practitioners are alerted to respond and resolve the problem. Otherwise, determine and resolve the cause of the alarm before resetting it. If the cause cannot be determined, or the resolution is outside your scope of knowledge or practice, alert the nurse or caregiver.

Remain calm. A hysterical clinician on top of the piercing sound of the alarm will only increase the patient's anxiety and exacerbate the problem. Talk calmly to the patient, help the patient to breathe less effortfully and in a more controlled manner, and calmly seek assistance from other professionals as necessary. Do not leave the patient to seek assistance. Instead remain by the patient's side, send someone else for assistance and be ready to give aid, such as manual ventilation, if needed.

Check the tubing and circuitry running from the patient to the ventilator and back. Do a systematic visual check of the connections, starting with the connection nearest the patient and working all the way to the ventilator and back again. Many times a disconnected tube is the cause of an alarm. Should you find separated tubing, reconnect it as firmly as possible and wait for the ventilator alarm to reset itself. If the alarm continues, seek out the next possible cause.

Maintain current CPR and artificial resuscitation certifications and be ready to manually ventilate the individual. If you cannot find and resolve the cause of the alarm and the patient appears to be in distress, seek immediate aid (in a hospital call for the respiratory therapist, nurse or physician; or dial 911 if you are working in an individual's home). Initiate artificial respiration or ventilation with a manual resuscitation bag (a bag that either fits over the patient's mouth or attaches to the artificial airway to provide emergency ventilation). Hook the manual resuscitation bag up to 100% oxygen and provide manual breaths until instructed to do otherwise by a physician or emergency medical professional.

Types of Alarms

The following are the general types of alarms present on most ventilators. Again, there may be some variation in the location and exact name of the alarm, depending on the model of ventilator. Several types of alarms may be triggered by the use of a speaking valve in-line with the ventilator. Do not assume that an alarm is caused by the speaking valve until you have ruled out other possible causes. Remember, the patient would not be on a ventilator if he or she could breathe adequately without it; therefore, a ventilator alarm may be signaling a potentially life-threatening problem.

High Pressure Limit Alarm

The high pressure limit alarm activates when a patient's peak inspiratory pressure (PIP) is exceeded. This means that greater than usual pressure is needed to provide the necessary tidal volume.

Typical causes: coughing, water buildup in the tubing, secretions partially blocking the tubing, kinked or occluded tubing (for example, from the tubing getting caught in the bedding or the patient accidentally or deliberately squeezing or chewing on the tubing).

Typical actions: If coughing appears to be the problem, wait for the patient to recover and see if alarm resets itself; if not, suction the patient's airway (see chapter 7). Do a systematic visual check of the tubing, looking for kinks. If a kink is found, straighten it and make sure no damage has been done to the tube, replacing the tube if necessary. If water buildup is visible in the tubing, drain the tube using the water traps or by disconnecting the tube and tipping it *away* from the patient. (If you are not careful, you may drain the condensation collected in the tube directly into the patient's airway.) If secretions are present, suction the patient's airway or replace the tube with a fresh one if it is occluded by secretions.

Low Pressure Limit Alarm

A sounding low pressure limit alarm indicates that the amount of pressure needed to deliver the tidal volume has dropped below normal limits.

Typical causes: disconnected tubing, leak in the circuitry system, leak around the tracheostomy cuff or complete deflation of the cuff, the use of a speaking valve in-line with the ventilator.

Typical actions: Systematically inspect for disconnected tubing and reconnect it; check all the connections for leaks, including those to the water traps, heater temperature probes, in-line suction catheter systems and the expiratory end of the circuit. Check the inflation of the cuff and insert more air if appropriate. Be careful not to overinflate the cuff, and check the pressure limit with respiratory staff. If the patient is using a speaking valve in-line with the ventilator, request that the low pressure limit be lowered, *but be sure to have it reset* when the speaking valve is removed. (Do not reinflate the cuff if the patient is using a speaking valve.)

Apnea Alarm

The apnea alarm sounds when no air movement is detected, indicating that the patient may have stopped breathing. Because CPAP and pressure support modes are based on the patient's spontaneous breathing cycles, the apnea alarm is critical. The ventilator will not take over breathing for the patient in these modes.

Typical causes: Disconnected tubing, a leak in the circuitry system or around the tracheostomy cuff, deflation of the cuff, the use of a speaking valve in-line with the ventilator, reduction or cessation of spontaneous breathing by the patient.

Typical actions: If the patient has slowed or stopped breathing but is alert (for example, holding his or her breath because of the new sensation of a speaking valve), cue the patient to breathe in and out, and remove the speaking valve if the patient does not respond. If the patient seems groggy or disoriented, attempt to rouse the person to see if this will reinitiate breathing. Seek assistance from other staff or dial 911 (depending on setting) if the patient is having difficulty breathing. Perform artificial respiration or manual ventilation with a manual resuscitation bag if necessary until assistance arrives. Check for disconnected tubing and reconnect it; also do a systematic visual check of all connections, including those to the water traps, heater temperature probes, in-line suction catheter systems, and the expiratory end of the circuit. Check the inflation of the cuff and insert more air if appropriate. Be careful not to overinflate the cuff, and check the pressure limit with respiratory staff. If the patient is not in respiratory distress and the cause is clearly use of a speaking valve in-line with the ventilator, request that the apnea alarm be disabled if possible. Be sure the alarm is re-enabled after removal of the speaking valve.

Low Exhaled Volume Alarm

The low exhaled volume alarm activates when the ventilator receives a lower return of tidal volume during the expiratory phase than was delivered to the patient in the inspiratory phase. The alarm sounds when the ventilator does not receive equal or nearly equal the tidal volume delivered; typically the alarm is set about 100 ml below the prescribed tidal volume.

Typical causes: disconnected tubing, leak in the circuitry system, use of a speaking valve in-line with the ventilator.

Typical actions: Check for disconnected tubing and reconnect it; also do a systematic visual check for leaks at all connections, including those to the water traps, heater temperature probes, in-line suction catheter systems, and the expiratory end of the circuit. If the alarm has been triggered by use of a speaking valve in-line with the ventilator, request that the exhaled volume alarm be lowered or disabled, being sure it is re-enabled after the speaking valve is removed.

Low PEEP/CPAP Alarm

This alarm sounds when the prescribed levels of positive end-expiratory pressure or continual positive airway pressure are not maintained. (That is, the pressure in the airway or alveoli drops below normal.)

Typical causes: disconnected tubing, leak in the circuitry, leak around the cuff.

Typical actions: Check for disconnected tubing and reconnect it; also do a systematic visual check for leaks at all connections, including those to the water traps, heater temperature probes, in-line suction catheter systems, and the expiratory end of the circuit. Check the cuff for proper inflation and insert more air into the cuff if appropriate.

Vocal Communication with a Ventilator

The nonvocal communication options discussed in chapter 4 are applicable to patients on a ventilator. The most widely used means of vocal communication for patients who are ventilated is a one-way speaking valve used in-line with the ventilator. Currently, the Passy-Muir Speaking Valves (PMVs) are the only type of speaking valves that can be used in-line with a ventilator (see figure 6.4) . The specific model of PMV valve selected depends on whether the ventilator tubing used is disposable or non-disposable. Disposable tubing requires the PMV 007 aqua-colored valve, while non-disposable tubing calls for the PMV 2000 clear valve or the 2001 purple valve. The patient can continue to use the same valve with a tracheostomy tube alone after being weaned from the ventilator.

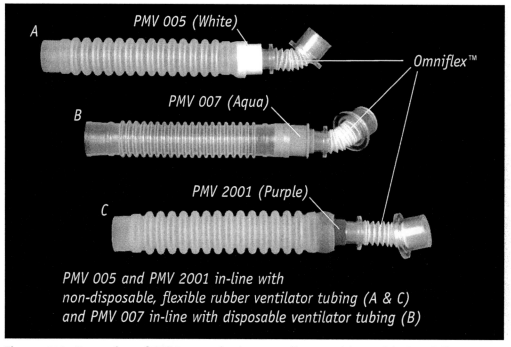

Figure 6.4. Examples of PMVs attached to ventilator tubing with Omni-flex. (Photo courtesy of Passy-Muir, Inc.)

For adult patients, there are three main reasons to introduce use of an in-line speaking valve. The first is improving communication. Although writing is an effective means of communication for patients with the literacy and fine motor skill to use it, many patients feel relieved to be able to communicate vocally again. The second is to improve the safety and efficiency of swallowing. As discussed in chapter 4, the speaking valve improves senses of taste and smell, normalizes subglottic pressure, and may help with secretion management and sensation, all of which contribute to safer and more efficient swallowing. The third reason is to assist with weaning from the ventilator. The use of the speaking valve in-line with the ventilator can help to improve oxygen saturation and provides for a stronger cough (which helps not only to clear secretions but also to strengthen musculature; Lichtmann et al. 1995). Also not to be discounted are the psychological benefits of improved communication and socialization, which may increase motivation.

The same reasons apply with infants and children as well. In fact, infants are never too young for a speaking valve trial, as long as they fit the criteria below. The use of an in-line speaking valve allows infants to develop speech and language skills by providing opportunities for cooing and babbling and the feedback of hearing their own voices. As well, an in-line speaking valve can promote a safer and more efficient swallow, enhance taste and smell and promote weaning, just as it does with adults.

■ Candidacy for Speaking Valve Trials

To be a candidate for a speaking valve, a patient must meet the following criteria. These criteria have already been presented in chapter 4, but they are reviewed here for your convenience. These criteria are only guidelines. For many patients, their success (or difficulty) using a speaking valve can be determined only with a trial. If you are uncertain whether a patient is a candidate, a short-term trial may be indicated.

1. The physician has signed an order or prescription authorizing the trial.

2. The upper airway must be free of obstructions or stenoses so that air can flow freely through the vocal cords for phonation and through the mouth for articulation. This may include obstruction caused by the tracheostomy tube itself. For example, a Shiley® #8 tracheostomy tube may fit snugly enough inside the trachea to prevent significant airflow around the tube and up into the glottis for phonation.

3. The patient must be able to tolerate cuff deflation.

4. The vocal cords must be functional to produce adequate phonation for speech. (Sometimes this cannot be determined until an actual trial with the valve.)

5. The patient must not be using the Bivona Fome-Cuf® tracheostomy tube. If the patient currently has this type of tube, ask the respiratory therapists and

pulmonologists about the possibility of changing the tracheostomy tube to another brand to enable vocal communication.

6. If the patient has excessive amounts of secretions that require frequent suctioning, management of the secretions should be addressed before a speaking valve is placed. The use of a Passy-Muir speaking valve has been documented to decrease the volume of secretions a patient produces (Lichtmann et al. 1995). Use of the PMV increases the management of secretions, helps to filter the inhaled air of dust, improves the strength of a cough and improves swallowing, all of which aid in secretion management.

7. The patient should be medically stable and should not have other pressing medical needs or complications. Remember that the speaking valve may increase the stress on the respiratory system. A related factor to consider is the percentage of oxygen the patient needs. Typically, patients who need more than 40 percent FiO_2 are not good candidates until their need for supplemental oxygen can be decreased. Discussion with the respiratory therapist or pulmonologist on your team can assist in that determination.

■ Ventilator Setting Adjustments

In order to accommodate the use of an in-line speaking valve, the ventilator settings must be adjusted. In most cases, the respiratory therapist or nurse should make these changes. After being fully trained by the appropriate professionals, however, the speech-language pathologist can, on occasion, make the necessary adjustments. If you ever do adjust any ventilator settings, be sure to return them to their original values after the speaking valve is removed. The following is a general description of the necessary adjustments to the ventilator settings. Again, do not attempt to make these adjustments yourself without consulting a physician, respiratory therapist or nurse, unless you have been properly trained.

Tidal volume. The placement of the speaking valve changes the direction of exhaled air. Instead of going back into the ventilator, the exhaled air is directed out through the pharynx. Due to this "loss" of exhaled air, the amount of air, or tidal volume, given may need to be increased. The increase should be such that the peak inspiratory pressure that was present before cuff deflation is re-established.

Positive end expiratory pressure (PEEP). If the ventilator is providing 5 cm H_2O or less of PEEP, the PEEP value should be eliminated to compensate for the pressure automatically provided by the PMV.

Alarm settings. Increasing the tidal volume may necessitate a higher ventilator pressure to deliver that air. If so, it is necessary to disable or adjust the peak inspiratory pressure alarm to avoid its being triggered unnecessarily. In addition, the escape of air through the pharynx is likely to trigger the low expiratory volume and apnea alarms. It may be necessary to adjust or disable these alarms as well.

Valve Placement

The speaking valve should be placed as close to the tracheostomy tube hub as possible. The farther the speaking valve is from the hub, the more resistance the patient has to overcome in order to phonate. Whenever possible, the speaking valve should be placed directly on the hub (see figure 6.5a). If an in-line suctioning unit is attached to the hub of the tracheostomy tube, the speaking valve can be connected to the side port with an adapter (usually a 15 x 22 mm "step-down" adapter) to prevent the suctioning catheter from damaging the speaking valve and the speaking valve from obstructing the ability to suction (see figure 6.5b).

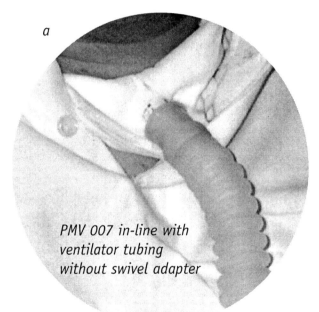

a

PMV 007 in-line with ventilator tubing without swivel adapter

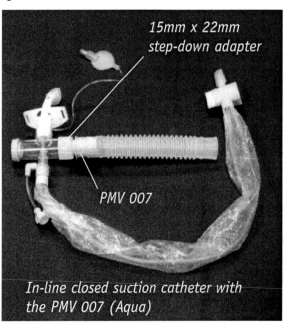

b

15mm x 22mm step-down adapter

PMV 007

In-line closed suction catheter with the PMV 007 (Aqua)

Figure 6.5. PMV attached in-line to a ventilator: (a) directly to the hub; and (b) with an in-line suctioning unit. (Photos courtesy of Passy-Muir, Inc.)

In-Line Speaking Valve Trial Flow Sheet

Patient: Patient ID:		Date:
Trach type/size: [ ] Cuff [ ] No cuff [ ] Fenestrated		Valve used:

Baseline ventilator settings (per respiratory therapist):

Precautions:

Changes to ventilator settings (per respiratory therapist):

Start time:		End time:
1. Baseline Measures	O_2: HR: RR: Color: Effort:	
2. Deflate cuff	Amount of air withdrawn: cc	
3. Suction trachea and oral cavity	Amount/color of secretions: Strength of cough:	
4. Turn off expiratory and apnea alarms		
5. Increase V_t if needed	New V_t:	
6. Place speaking valve	Time:	
7. Suction orally	Secretions:	
8. Repeat measures	O_2: HR: RR: Color: Effort:	
9. Cue voicing	Vocal quality:	
10. Repeat measures	O_2: HR: RR: Color: Effort:	
11. Remove valve	Time:	
12. Return settings/alarms to original values		
13. Inflate cuff	Amount of air replaced: cc	
14. Repeat measures	O_2: HR: RR: Color: Effort:	

Comments:

Speech-language pathologist:

Respiratory therapist:

Physician:

Tracheostomy Tubes and Ventilator Dependence in Adults and Children—VanDahm and Sparks-Walsh

© 2002 by PRO-ED, Inc.

Protocol for a Trial of the PMV In-line with a Ventilator

Upon receipt of the physician's order or prescription, clinical trials of the PMV in-line with the ventilator should be conducted in the following manner. (The form on page 114 may be copied and used for recording necessary information throughout the speaking valve trial.)

1. Educate the patient and family (if applicable) about the speaking valve.

2. Obtain baseline measures of oxygen saturation, heart rate, respiratory rate, tidal volume and PIP.

3. Suction the individual's mouth and trachea as needed.

4. Deflate the tracheostomy cuff or request that the appropriate staff member do so. In most facilities the respiratory or nursing staff maintains an exact measure of cuff pressure. Be sure to record how much air is withdrawn from the cuff to fully deflate it, so you can reinflate the cuff with exactly the same amount of air at the end of the trial. (Most infant and pediatric tracheostomy tubes are not cuffed. In that case, this step may be skipped.)

5. Disable or adjust expiratory and apnea alarms (usually with the assistance of nursing or respiratory professionals).

6. Turn off or adjust the PEEP settings (usually with the assistance of nursing or respiratory professionals).

7. Increase tidal volume if necessary (usually with the assistance of nursing or respiratory professionals).

8. Attach the speaking valve in-line with the ventilator.

9. Monitor the individual's response, including oxygen saturation level, respiratory rate, heart rate and skin coloring.

10. Cue the individual to begin vocalizing. Try beginning with rote speech such as counting or naming days of the week or months of the year. This helps the person to focus on vocalization rather than the content of the message. With children, focus on play and developmental sounds. Infants may begin crying and first achieve vocalization that way. Comfort the infant or child, redirect attention away from the changes in breathing and focus on play.

11. Provide visual cues on the inspiratory and expiratory cycles, if needed, to help the person learn to time vocalization to the expiratory phase. Many people require a little time to adjust to speaking in time with the cycles of the ventilator, rather than being able to take a breath at will and continue speaking.

12. Continue practicing speech while monitoring the person for signs of respiratory distress (see page 71 for signs of respiratory distress in adults and page 75 for additional signs in children). Terminate the trial immediately, remove the

speaking valve, and restore ventilator and cuff settings if the individual becomes groggy or shows other signs of inadequate oxygenation.

13. When the trial is complete, remove the speaking valve.

14. Return the ventilator settings and alarms to their previous settings.

15. Reinflate the cuff with the specified amount of air.

16. Monitor the individual's oxygenation level, respiratory rate, heart rate and appearance.

Initial trials may last anywhere from a few seconds to a few hours. Until the patient has demonstrated successful use and tolerance of the speaking valve over several occasions, however, he or she should never be left unattended with the valve in-line. Successful use and tolerance is demonstrated by maintenance of adequate oxygenation saturation levels, ease of breathing, functional vocal quality, stable heart rate and no feelings of discomfort.

Recent literature has suggested an alternative to using a speaking valve in-line for vocal communication. In collaborative studies conducted by the University of Arizona and Harvard Medical School, researchers have changed the ventilator settings to support speech through a fenestrated tracheostomy tube or deflated tracheostomy cuff. This procedure has the advantage that an individual on a positive pressure ventilator can vocalize on both inspiratory and expiratory cycles. (Air flowing either direction will escape through the fenestrations or deflated cuff and up through the glottis, allowing for phonation.) Extending the inspiratory time of the ventilator setting (increasing the I:E ratio such that the inspiratory cycle is equal to or greater than the expiratory cycle), will increase speaking time, allowing the patient to speak in longer phrases and have fewer silences in conversation. The second ventilator change is to add a positive end-expiratory pressure (or PEEP), ranging from an additional 5 to 10 cm H_2O. Thus the speaking time during the expiratory phase can be prolonged as well. Studies have shown that this type of ventilator-supported speech is more fluent and less variable in loudness than speech produced by deflating the cuff without making these ventilatory changes (Hoit 1997). Some issues raised in these studies that may require further investigation are (1) the consequences of higher amounts of air being diverted to the larynx for sustained speech instead of being used in the lungs, (2) the risk of breath stacking and its consequences if limiting the expiratory cycle does not allow sufficient time to fully expire each breath, and (3) the increased risk of barotraumas due to higher levels of PEEP increasing intrathoracic pressure.

Ventilators and Swallowing

Swallowing while on a ventilator is a tricky business. Many professionals mistakenly believe that since the cuff is inflated, the airway is protected and swallowing safety is not an issue. As you will recall from chapter 5, any material that reaches the level of the cuff has already been aspirated and it is important to make this point to your colleagues. On the other hand, patients who are on long-term ventilator support should not be excluded from swallowing evaluations and trials.

Ventilator-dependent individuals who wish to eat and drink safely must meet certain criteria. First, learning the necessary strategy requires some cognitive ability. Patients who cannot follow commands or give accurate feedback are probably not appropriate candidates for dysphagia therapy.

Second, the ventilator creates artificial pressures and airflow in the pharynx and trachea. Not only are normal subglottic pressures significantly disrupted simply by the placement of the tracheostomy tube, but the pressures and air volumes created by the ventilator to support air exchange augment the changes in subglottic pressures. Even with the cuff inflated, air can leak around the cuff and enter the pharynx. With the cuff deflated, large volumes of air escape through the mouth and nose, making it very difficult to hold one's breath during a swallow in order to protect the airway and prevent the bolus from being involuntarily expelled out the nose or mouth. On the other hand, repeated swallowing with the cuff inflated can lead to tracheal tissue damage and even a tracheoesophageal fistula due to the friction of the cuff rubbing against the tracheal wall with every swallow.

Use of the in-line speaking valve during a swallowing assessment is recommended if possible. The use of an in-line speaking valve can improve the swallowing function of an individual on a ventilator, for the same reasons as with someone who is tracheostomized but not ventilated. The valve may return pharyngeal pressure to a more normal level, enabling the individual to cough more effectively. Improved pharyngeal and laryngeal sensation may help to reduce pooling in the pharynx because the individual can sense the pooled material and cough or swallow to clear it. Improved senses of taste and smell increase the motivation to eat. Finally, deflation of the cuff usually decreases the tethering effect of the artificial airway on the larynx, possibly increasing laryngeal elevation. All of these effects can create a safer and more efficient swallow.

Assessments such as the modified barium swallow study (MBS), modified Evan's blue dye test and fiberoptic endoscopic evaluation of swallowing (FEES®) can be performed with the speaking valve in-line with the ventilator. Procedures for each of these tests are the same as discussed in chapter 5 (see pages 87-95) and will not be repeated here. Note, however, that it is important to have either a respiratory therapist or nurse deflate the cuff before suctioning to allow any aspirated material that may have pooled above the cuff to fall into the trachea for detection during suctioning. Otherwise a false negative response may be obtained.

Sometimes it may be necessary to evaluate the individual's swallow without the speaking valve in place. In such a case, it is very important to deflate the cuff and suction out any material that may have been aspirated and pooled above the cuff. Do this while following the blue dye protocol described in chapter 5 (page 87).

Some amount of coaching and training will be necessary before and during the swallowing assessment, depending on the patient and the nature of the changes made to the ventilator settings to accommodate the in-line speaking valve. If the tidal volume was increased, a large volume of air may escape through the mouth during every exhalation. If so, the individual may need to practice redirecting the air through the nose. Learning to close the mouth and direct the exhaled air through the nose will allow the patient time to collect and organize the bolus in the oral cavity prior to swallowing. Because the patient has become accustomed to breathing exclusively through the tracheostomy tube prior to speaking valve use, your initial swallowing goals may involve the patient adjusting to the new sensations of airflow through the oral cavity and gaining voluntary control of the velum in order to time velar movements to the cycles of the ventilator.

Given the volume of air and the pressure exerted by the ventilator, many patients find it very difficult to hold their breath during the exhalation phase and stop the flow of air from entering the pharynx so that they can swallow. In this case, the patient should also practice timing the swallow to coincide with the inspiratory phase of the ventilator prior to a swallowing trial. To help patients learn to recognize the initiation and conclusion of the inspiration and expiration cycles, cue them to notice the change in oral and pharyngeal sensations, to hear the ventilator sounds associated with each cycle and even to look at the lights on the face of the ventilator. Once patients can recognize the end of the exhalation and inhalation phases, and have demonstrated the ability to swallow their own saliva safely and efficiently, food trials with small boluses can begin.

Throughout the swallowing trials, be sure to monitor oxygen saturation, heart rate and skin color (as described in chapter 2, pages 24-28), the ability to cough effectively and vocal quality for signs of respiratory difficulty. After presentation of each texture and upon completion of the trials, be sure to suction the patient's trachea. If the boluses have been dyed blue, be sure to observe the suctioning catheter for traces of blue (but bear in mind that the absence of blue does not guarantee the absence of aspiration).

Ventilators and the Pediatric Population

Infants and children respond to changes differently than adults do. It is very important that we take these sensitivities seriously and approach the treatment of a child on a ventilator with extra care and compassion. For children, especially those who were vocal before the incident that required ventilation, the inability to vocalize, communicate or eat as they used to do can be a critical and very frightening psychological concern.

Speaking Valve Trials

As discussed in chapter 4, it is never too early to start speaking valve trials with little ones (barring significant medical complications), so as to minimize the disruption to their speech and language development. Infants who have been ventilator-dependent since birth may not recognize their own voices or their power to use the voice as a tool for communication. Infants who are able to use speaking valves in-line have opportunities to hear their own voices and the consequences of using the voice, and are able to develop verbal skills of cooing, babbling and phoneme development as they would if the need for ventilation were not there (see figure 6.6).

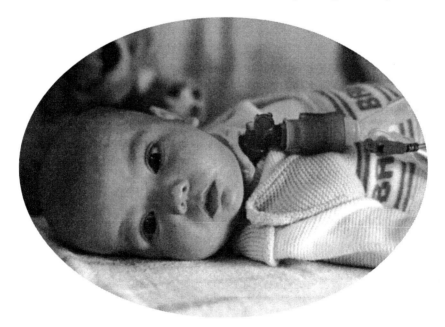

Figure 6.6. Infant with PMV in-line with a ventilator. (Photo courtesy of Passy-Muir, Inc.)

As discussed in chapter 2, it is important to do a thorough chart review to determine whether an infant or child is an appropriate candidate for an in-line speaking valve. Contraindications to the use of a speaking valve include tracheal stenosis, tracheomalacia (softening or collapse of the tracheal cartilage), paralysis of the vocal cords in the adducted position, copious or thick secretions, a tracheostomy tube that fits snugly inside the trachea and doesn't allow airflow around it, medical instability and a foam-filled tracheostomy cuff. Many of these problems are not discovered until the initial speaking valve trial, however, so in questionable cases, discussion with the primary care physician before a speaking valve trial is recommended. If problems become apparent during the trial, you may recommend that the physician conduct further investigation and diagnostic procedures.

Some children become very guarded when coping with the changes in their breathing and their inability to speak; realizing that the speaking valve can return their ability to communicate vocally can be a great relief for them. That the speaking valve is the means by which communication is achieved must be reinforced, and use of the valve rewarded, as often as possible during the treatment sessions. For example, explaining the use of the speaking valve, letting the child hold the valve prior to placement and even drawing designs on it may lessen the child's anxiety about using it. If possible, arrange for a family member, familiar caretaker or a child life specialist to be present to hold and reassure the child (this adult can also be useful for modeling vocalizations). Make eye contact frequently and provide reassuring touch often.

In-line speaking valve trials with children are similar to those with adults, but, of course, with utterances and interactions that are age appropriate (see figure 6.7). Changes in ventilator settings may or may not be indicated, depending on the individual child. Seek the advice of the primary care physician or a respiratory specialist.

As with an adult, you will take baseline measurements of oxygen saturation, heart rate, peak inspiratory pressure and tidal volumes prior to the speaking trials (see page 114). However, infants and children differ significantly from adults in their response to respiratory changes. Be aware that they may "crash," or experience sudden respiratory distress. It is important to recognize signs of respiratory decline quickly and take steps to prevent the child from reaching respiratory failure. Warning signs are increased respiratory rate, decreasing oxygenation, increased heart rate, sudden restlessness, flaring of the nares, mottling of the skin (in which the superficial veins begin to show more prominently) and decreasing alertness. Immediately remove the valve, reset the ventilator, and monitor the child.

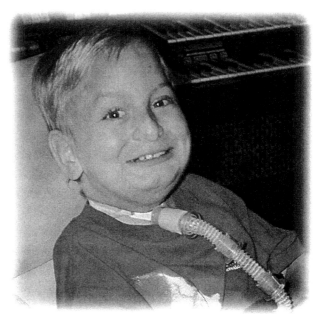

Figure 6.7. Child with PMV in-line with a ventilator. (Photo courtesy of Passy-Muir, Inc.)

Mechanical Ventilation

▓ In-line Swallowing Trials

Whether an infant can swallow safely while on a ventilator is a tough determination. Because infants take liquids through their bottles with an almost constant flow, and because their cognitive abilities are still developing, you should be very careful when initiating feeding trials. Since infants typically breathe in and out through the nose while swallowing, they probably will not need to learn to coordinate swallowing with the ventilator cycles. The ability to close the glottis against the ventilator breaths and protect the airway from aspiration is a greater concern. Blue dye trials are a relatively easy method of assessment if you keep in mind their limitations: too much blue dye can cause an upset stomach for infants and children and the absence of blue secretions does not guarantee that no aspiration is occurring. The protocol for such trials is the same as for adults (see pages 88-89).

Another important consideration is the relationship between dysphagia and the length of time a premature infant is ventilated. A study at Northeast Louisiana University found that premature infants ventilated for fourteen to twenty-one days had a higher incidence of feeding and swallowing disorders. In addition, this group (as compared to infants with shorter-term ventilation or no ventilation) experienced more episodes of pneumonia and greater oral aversion (Oliver et al. 1998).

Conclusion

Working with ventilator-dependent patients can be an intimidating experience. However, an understanding of the modes of ventilation and the differences between controlled ventilation versus spontaneous ventilation and between the various modes in these categories will be of great benefit when developing functional treatment plans. Familiarity with the parameters of ventilator settings (such as tidal volume, rate, oxygen percentage and peak inspiratory pressure) and an understanding of the nature of ventilator alarms and how to problem-solve their causes will help lessen your anxiety and help you project an attitude of confidence to the patient. Building a strong working relationship with other health care practitioners, particularly respiratory specialists, is tremendously valuable. Use of a speaking valve in-line with the ventilator can enable patients of all ages to communicate vocally and may also improve the safety and efficiency of their swallowing. You have the opportunity to contribute significantly to the quality of life of those individuals who need the assistance of a ventilator.

Chapter 7

Tracheostomy Care and Hygiene Issues

It should be apparent by now that speech-language pathologists play a very important role in assisting adults and children with a tracheostomy tube or on a ventilator to achieve effective communication and safe swallowing. This chapter presents peripheral issues that may arise throughout a speech-language pathologist's involvement in a case, depending on the facility and its policies.

Tracheostomy Care

For a person with a tracheostomy tube, maintaining an open airway is of utmost importance. In the medical setting, tracheostomy care is typically carried out by nursing staff or respiratory therapists. It is certainly within the speech-language pathologist's scope of practice to emphasize the importance of tracheostomy hygiene to patients, family members and caregivers. Adults and older children can learn to perform their own tracheostomy care to the extent they are able. Training patients to remove their own inner cannula for cleaning or replacement and to care for the tracheostoma site promotes their independence and active participation in their medical care. Typically, respiratory therapists or nurses provide this training, although reinforcement, encouragement and further education from the speech-language pathologist is always beneficial.

A tracheostomy tube is cleaned by removing the inner cannula and placing it in a solution of hydrogen peroxide (kits are available; see figure 7.1, page 124). A thin wire brush is inserted into the inner cannula to assist in removing thickened, dried secretions. After cleaning, the inner cannula is rinsed with a saline solution, allowed to dry and replaced within the outer cannula.

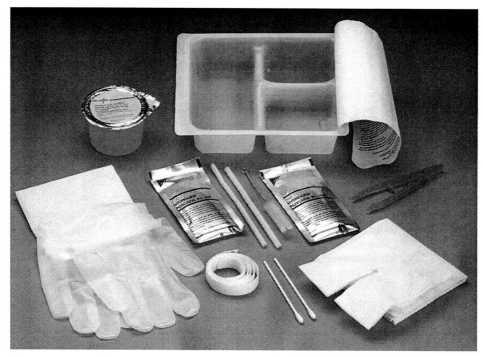

Figure 7.1 Tracheostomy cleaning kit. (Courtesy of Medline Industries, Inc.)

Speaking Valve Care

Standard cleaning protocols vary depending on the manufacturer and the specific product. Cleaning and care guidelines are typically packaged with the valve. Please familiarize yourself, the patient and family members with them.

Maintaining a Patent Airway

Coughing is the natural means of clearing the airway of secretions. Many adults and children are not able to cough effectively to expectorate their secretions or mucus. These patients require periodic suctioning to clear the airway. Suctioning is an invasive technique used only when the patient is unable to clear the airway by coughing, and its use and frequency typically will be prescribed by the physician. There are three reasons for suctioning: (1) to maintain a patent airway by reducing secretion buildup, (2) to stimulate a deeper and more effective cough, and (3) to remove aspirated material. Suctioning should be a quick procedure; the total time from insertion to withdrawal of the suctioning catheter should not exceed about fifteen seconds.

Many facilities utilize one or more of the suctioning techniques described below. The following general descriptions will orient you to the basic procedure and serve as a reminder if you suction patients only infrequently. We recommend that speech-language pathologists be trained to suction both in-line and by sterile procedure. This training should be provided by competent healthcare professionals and according to the policies and procedures of your facility or organization.

Sterile suctioning: In sterile suctioning, you begin by creating and maintaining a sterile field and putting on sterile gloves in a sterile manner (see figure 7.2). After attaching the sterile suction catheter to the suctioning unit, insert the suction catheter (with the suction port open) into the area to be suctioned—the tracheostomy tube, nasal cavity or oral cavity. Advance it the appropriate distance, either to a specific measurement marked on the catheter or until a cough is elicited. In some cases you may need to apply a saline wash. Then occlude the suction port with a gloved index finger (see figure 7.3) and slowly withdraw the catheter while rolling it between your fingers. If necessary, flush the catheter with saline solution to clear it of mucus. If it is necessary to suction the patient a second time, allow a brief rest period between suctioning intervals, while maintaining a sterile field. Dispose of the suctioning equipment according to the guidelines of your facility.

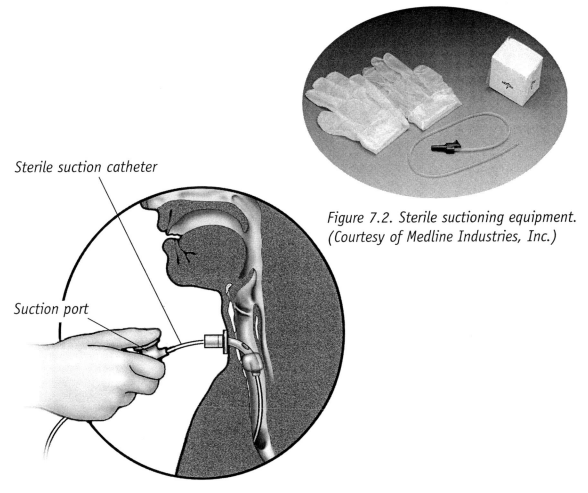

Figure 7.2. Sterile suctioning equipment. (Courtesy of Medline Industries, Inc.)

Figure 7.3. Sterile suctioning through a tracheostomy tube.

Suctioning through a nasal trumpet: A nasal trumpet is used to protect the mucosal lining of the nasal cavity when frequent nasal suctioning is necessary (see figure 7.4). The basic procedure is the same as for sterile suctioning, but the suctioning catheter is passed through a nasal trumpet that directs it into the pharynx and then down to the trachea for suctioning. (Do not confuse a nasal trumpet with a nasal endotracheal tube, a very different piece of equipment.) In most facilities, personnel other than SLPs will do suctioning through a nasal trumpet.

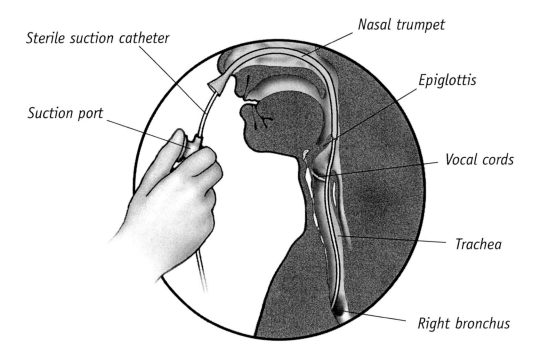

Figure 7.4. Sterile suctioning through a nasal trumpet.

In-line (or closed) suctioning: In-line suctioning refers to a completely self-contained, sterile suction unit that attaches directly to the tracheostomy tube and can remain in place for up to forty-eight hours before being replaced (rather than being discarded after each suctioning episode). The suction catheter is covered with plastic to prevent contact with outside elements and maintain sterility (see figure 7.5). Recall from chapter 6 that a Passy-Muir speaking valve can remain in place during in-line suctioning if the proper adapter is used.

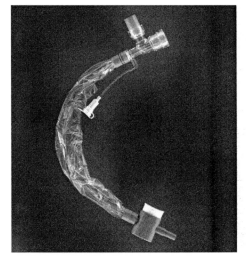

Figure 7.5. In-line suctioning unit. (Courtesy of Kimberly-Clark/Ballard Medical)

Oral suctioning: Oral suctioning is a less invasive procedure that may be necessary to assist a patient who has difficulty with saliva management. The patient may perform oral suctioning independently, or family members or staff members may assist if needed. Oral suctioning may be necessary during a swallowing trial if the patient has difficulty swallowing a particular food or liquid. The speech-language pathologist should suction the patient promptly to remove the material from the oral cavity before it can be aspirated. Yankauer tips are commonly used for oral suctioning for adults (see figure 7.6); smaller versions, sometimes referred to as tonsil tips, can be used with infants and children.

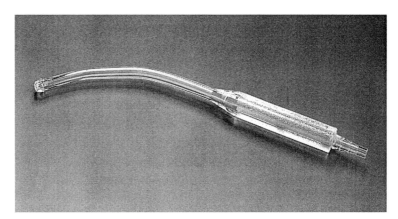

Figure 7.6. Yankauer suction tip. (Courtesy of Medline Industries, Inc.)

Because proper suctioning technique promotes patient safety and reduces trauma to the patient, it is imperative that the practitioner be properly trained before attempting any type of suctioning procedure. Depending on the facility, the speech-language pathologist (among others) may or may not be trained to perform this task. In some facilities, speech-language pathologists learn to perform only in-line suctioning whereas in others they learn both in-line and sterile suctioning. The American Speech-Language-Hearing Association (ASHA) supports the involvement of speech-language pathologists in suctioning, provided they have been adequately trained and deemed competent to do so (ASHA 1996). The ASHA position statement is available to members on-line at ASHA's web site or by contacting the association.

Oral Hygiene

To reduce the risk of infection from aspirated secretions, it is important to encourage the patient (or caregivers) to maintain good oral hygiene. Many different products are commercially available for this purpose. The most popular and best-known device is an oral swab, commonly marketed under the brand name Toothette®. This is a sponge attached to a stick, which can be moistened and used to clean oral structures. There is also a similar device that can be attached to a suctioning unit, to assist in managing excess liquid and secretions (see figure 7.7, page 128). Patients who are alert and able to move may be able to "swish and spit"; that is, to rinse the oral cavity with mouthwash and spit it out into a basin without swallowing.

Recall from chapter 5, however, that it is important to postpone oral care when doing a modified Evan's blue dye test for secretion management. The blue dye is placed directly on the patient's tongue and oral care will remove it, negating the evaluation. Be certain to notify the nursing staff to suspend oral care and indicate how much time should pass before it may be resumed, usually twenty-four hours.

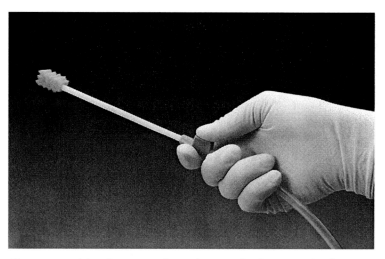

Figure 7.7. Toothette oral swab attached to suctioning attachment port. (Courtesy of Sage Products, Inc., Cary, IL)

Supplies to Keep Readily Available

The following is a list of equipment and supplies that you should have on hand if you work with adults or children who require tracheostomy tubes or ventilators. For speech-language pathologists who are itinerant or provide in-home care, it is particularly important to prepare and maintain a kit of supplies. It is also advisable to have extras of any supplies that the patient or family members are trained to use, so you can leave a supply with them. Some items are patient-specific, meaning that they can be used for only one patient and must be discarded when that person no longer has a need for them. Consult the vendor list in Appendix B for sources to purchase necessary equipment.

■ Personal Protective Equipment

For your own protection as well as that of your clients, you should always wear personal protective equipment when providing therapy to individuals who are tracheotomized, especially if they are hospitalized or carrying an infection (see figure 7.8). Protective equipment is of the utmost importance when evaluating or treating an individual with an antibiotic-resistant respiratory infection, such as MRSA (methicillin-resistant staphylococcus aureus), VRE (vancomycin-resistant enterococci), or ARSA (antibiotic-resistant staphylococcus aureus). Hospitals have strict protocols regarding precautions to be taken when working with a patient who has an infectious disease.

Face mask. Wear a face mask to protect your face from expectorated mucus or secre-

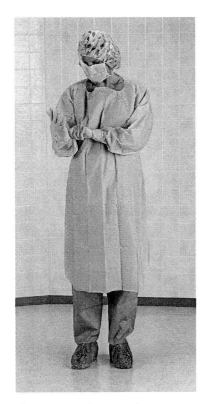

Figure 7.8. Personal protection equipment. (Courtesy of Medline Industries, Inc.)

◼ Other Supplies

Sterile suction kits. These kits are available in various sizes for pediatric and adult patients. While most individuals have their own supplies at home, it may be beneficial to have a few on hand for backup. Common sizes are 12–14 French diameter for adults, 8–10 French diameter for children and 6–8 French diameter for infants.

tions and from other airborne particulates. A face mask also protects the patient from catching any illness you may be incubating (such as a cold).

Gloves. Wear examination gloves to protect yourself from any infection the patient may have and to ensure that you do not transmit any disease or infection to the patient. Gloves also protect against blood-borne pathogens (see figure 7.9).

Gown. Wearing a gown protects your clothing from expectorated mucus or secretions and further protects against cross-contamination between clients.

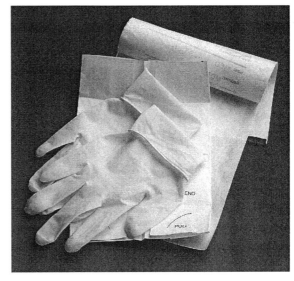

Figure 7.9. Sterile examination gloves. (Courtesy of Medline Industries, Inc.)

Penlight. A penlight is useful for looking into the tracheostomy tube and assessing the patency of the airway. It is also helpful when performing oral hygiene or for patient education regarding oral hygiene or stoma care.

Tracheostomy tube cleaning kits. Tracheostomy tube cleaning kits are available from a variety of sources. Most kits contain everything necessary for cleaning. Detailed instructions are also included.

Speaking valves. Having a speaking valve readily available is useful when a patient is attempting to use a valve for the first time. Valves are patient-specific and can be expensive. If only one type of speaking valve can be purchased, we recommend the Passy-Muir Tracheostomy Speaking Valve because it can be used either with or without a ventilator. After the patient's ability to use a valve has been established, you can assist the patient, family or physician in purchasing the best model of valve. Most healthcare facilities have a supply of valves on hand, but speech-language pathologists working outside medical facilities may need to assist their clients in obtaining the necessary valves. The cost may be covered by the individual's insurance if a physician writes a prescription for a specific valve. It is useful to have a small supply of valves available for use in the interim before the patient's permanent valve arrives. If possible, charge the individual for the valve you supply and recommend that the patient save it as a backup in case the permanent valve becomes lost or broken.

Disposable syringes. Syringes are necessary for inflating and deflating the tracheostomy tube cuff. A fresh syringe should be used with every patient.

Portable pulse oximeter. An oximeter is useful for monitoring oxygen saturation levels during speaking valve or swallowing trials and when monitoring a patient's tolerance for therapy (see figure 7.10).

Different consistencies and textures of food and liquid. Having a variety of foods and liquids available is necessary for proper evaluation of swallowing.

Portable suctioning machine. An adult or child who returns home from the hospital with a tracheostomy tube or ventilator will have to purchase a portable suctioning unit. This expense is covered by most insurance companies. If you work with this population frequently, you may wish to purchase one to have as a backup.

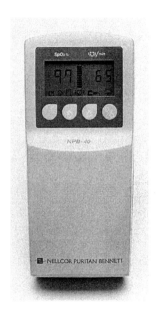

Figure 7.10. Portable pulse oximeter. (Reprinted by permission of Nellcor Puritan Bennett, Inc., Pleasanton, CA.)

Pictures or diagrams for patient education. We find it useful to have the following types of pictures to show when educating a patient or family members:

- anatomical placement of tracheostomy tube

- speaking valve function

- swallowing with an inflated tracheostomy tube cuff

Several reproducible illustrations for patient and family education are provided in Appendix C (page 143).

Other materials for patient education. It is useful to have informational brochures and samples of speaking valves and tracheostomy tubes available to show when explaining these devices and how they may affect speech or swallowing.

Blue dye. Blue or green dye is necessary for performing blue dye swallowing assessments. For each client, either purchase or ask the individual to purchase a bottle of household food coloring (preferably with preservatives, if available). Have the client store his or her personal bottle in the refrigerator for use in therapy.

Conclusion

Speech-language pathologists have a duty to maintain current education and training on all aspects of the treatment of adults and children with tracheostomy tubes or ventilators. A general understanding of many areas improves our ability to work collaboratively with other team members and provide integrated care to the patient. We also have a responsibility to continue to increase our knowledge and stay current with new developments and techniques through continuing education. There may be times when we are asked to perform skills that fall outside the requirements for the American-Speech-Language-Hearing Association Certification of Clinical Competency (CCC-SLP). Seek authorization and appropriate training from your facility and do not hesitate to seek the assistance of the appropriate professionals whenever questions arise about issues outside your area of expertise.

Appendix A:

Clinical Values and Measurements Associated with Patient Monitoring and Care

Apgar Score*

Sign	Score		
	0	1	2
Appearance	Blue or pale	Blue extremities	Pink
Pulse	Absent	Less than 100/min.	More than 100/min.
Grimace	No response	Grimace	Cough or sneeze
Activity	Limp	Some flexion	Active
Respiration	Absent	Slow/irregular	Good/crying
*Calculated at one and five minutes after delivery.			

Average Readings

Oxygen saturation (SaO_2):   90–100%
Peripheral arterial oxygenation (PaO_2):   80–100 mm Hg
Peripheral arterial carbon dioxide ($PaCO_2$):   35–45 mm Hg
Bicarbonate level (HCO_3):   23–25 mEq/l
Blood acidity (pH):   7.35–7.45
Base excess: 0 +/- 2 mEq/l

Average Blood Pressure

Infants: 80/40 mm Hg
Children: 100/60 mm Hg
Adults: 120/80 mm Hg

Average Pulse/Heart Rate

Infants: 120–160
Children: 80–140
Young adults: 75–100
Adults: 60–100

Average Respiratory Rate

Infants: 60–80 bpm
Children: 30–40 bpm
Adults: 14–20 bpm

Typical Ventilator Settings and Pulmonary Measures

Typical sensitivity value: -2 cm H_2O

Typical PEEP value: 2–5 cm H_2O

Percentage oxygen in room air: 21% O_2

I:E (inspiration:expiration) ratio: 1:2 seconds

(Infants and children have shorter inspiratory and expiratory times of .3 and .6 seconds, respectively, but the ratio remains 1:2.)

Standard Sterile Suction Tube Diameters

Infants: 6–8 French

Children: 8–10 French

Adults: 12–14 French

Appendix B:
Vendor List

AbleNet, Inc.
1081 Tenth Ave., S.E.
Minneapolis, MN 55414-1312
(800) 322-0956
www.ablenetinc.com
(augmentative/alternative communication devices)

Advanced Multimedia Devices, Inc. (AMDI)
31 Watermill Lane
Great Neck, NY 11021
(888) 353-AMDI
www.amdi.net
(augmentative/alternative communication devices)

Allegiance Healthcare Corporation
1430 Waukegan Road
McGaw Park, IL 60085-6787
(800) 964-5227
www.allegiance.net/home.asp
(Omni-flex connectors)

American Speech-Language-Hearing Association (ASHA)
10801 Rockville Pike
Rockville, MD 20852
(800) 638-8255
www.professional.asha.org
www.asha.org

Assistive Technology, Inc.
7 Wells Avenue
Newton, MA 02459
(800) 793-9227
www.assistivetech.com
(augmentative/alternative communication devices)

Ballard Medical Products
Kimberly-Clark (parent company)
12050 S. Lone Peak Parkway
Draper, UT 84020
(801) 572-6800
www.bmed.com
(15 mm x 22 mm step-down adapters, in-line sterile suction units)

Bayer Incorporated
Diagnostics Division
Elkhart, IN 46515
www.bayer.com
(Glucofilm® Test Strips)

Bivona Medical Technologies
28085 Ashley Circle, Suite 201A
Libertyville, IL 60048
(847) 549-0857
www.bivona.com
(Bivona Fome-Cuf® and Aire-Cuf® tracheostomy tubes, Bivona talking tracheostomy tube, endotracheal tubes)

Boston Medical Technologies
607 North Avenue, Suite 15
Wakefield, MA 01880
(877) 626-7267
www.bosmedtech.com
(Montgomery® speaking valve)

Imaginart International, Inc.
307 Arizona Street
Bisbee, AZ 85603
(800) 828-1376
www.imaginartonline.com
(augmentative/alternative communication aids)

Interactive Therapeutics, Inc.
P.O. Box 1805
Stow, OH 44224-0805
(800) 253-5111
www.interactivetherapy.com
(augmentative/alternative communication devices)

Kay Elemetrics Corporation
2 Bridgewater Lane
Lincoln Park, NJ 07035
(973) 628-6200
www.kayelemetrics.com
(Swallowing workstation [FEES®])

Nellcor Puritan-Bennett
Mallinckrodt (parent company)
675 McDonnell Blvd.
Hazelwood, MO 63042
(800) 634-1515
www.mallinckrodt.com
(Shiley® Phonate speaking valve, Shiley® tracheostomy tubes, tracheostomy tube neck
strap, nasal and oral endotracheal tubes, pulse oximeters and sensors, ventilators and
ventilator tubing, manual resuscitation bags, heat-moisture exchange devices)

Medline, Inc.
One Medline Place
Mundelein, IL 60060
1-800-MEDLINE
www.medline.com
(personal protective equipment, sterile suction kits, tracheostomy cleaning kits,
Yankauer suction tips, tracheostomy tube masks)

Passy-Muir, Inc.
PMB 273
4521 Campus Dr.
Irvine, CA 92612
(800) 634-5397
www.passy-muir.com
(Passy-Muir speaking valves and accessories, educational information)

Pilling Surgical
Suite 200
200 Precision Road
Horsham, PA 19044
(800) 523-6507
www.pillingsurgical.com
(Jackson metal tracheostomy tubes, Tucker valve, Shikani-French speaking valve)

Prentke Romich Company
1022 Heyl Rd.
Wooster, OH 44691
(800) 262-1984
www.prentrom.com
(augmentative/alternative communication devices)

Pulmonetic Systems, Inc.
930 South Mount Vernon Avenue, Suite 100
Colton, CA 92324
(800) 754-1914 or (909) 783-2280
www.pulmonetic.com
(LTV 900, LTV 950, LTV 1000 and accessories)

Sage Products, Inc.
3909 Three Oaks Road
Cary, IL 60013
(800) 323-2220
www.sageproducts.com
(Toothettes with or without suction attachment)

Dynavox Systems, Inc.
2100 Wharton Street, Suite 400
Pittsburgh, PA 15203
(800) 344-1778
(augmentative/alternative communication devices)

Portex, Inc.
10 Bowman Dr.
Keene, NH 03431
(800) 258-5361
www.portexusa.com
(in-line suction units, Per-fit percutaneous dilational tracheostomy kit, manual resuscitation bags, 15 mm endotracheal tube connectors for using Passy-Muir speaking valve with Jackson tracheostomy tubes, Orator speaking valve with Blue line Ultra tracheostomy tube kit, Portex talking tracheostomy tube)

Zygo Industries, Inc.
P.O. Box 1008
Portland, OR 97207-1008
(800) 234-6006
www.zygo-usa.com
(augmentative/alternative communication devices)

Appendix C:
Patient and Family Education Pages

Instructions

The following handouts are included for patient and family education. We have provided space to allow clinicians flexibility in responding to individual client needs. Each reproducible page has one or more illustrations and space to write specific instructions relevant to individual patient/family education. By selecting certain illustrations and creating a client-specific manual of educational handouts, clinicians can maximize treatment goals and promote a safe environment for each client's progress.

Tracheostomy Tube Placement

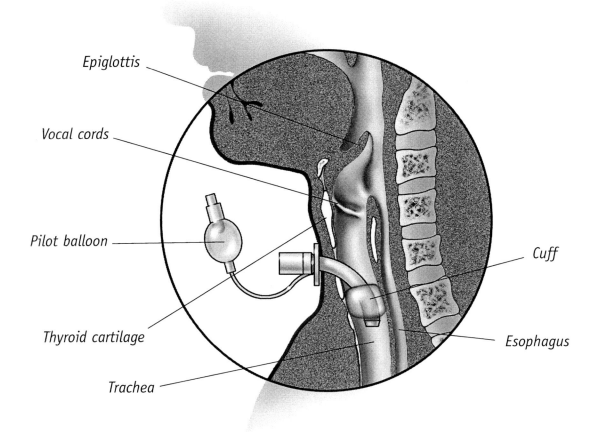

Epiglottis

Vocal cords

Pilot balloon

Thyroid cartilage

Trachea

Cuff

Esophagus

Comments and Instructions:

_____

_____

_____

_____

_____

_____

_____

_____

_____

_____

_____

_____

_____

_____

Adult and Child Airways

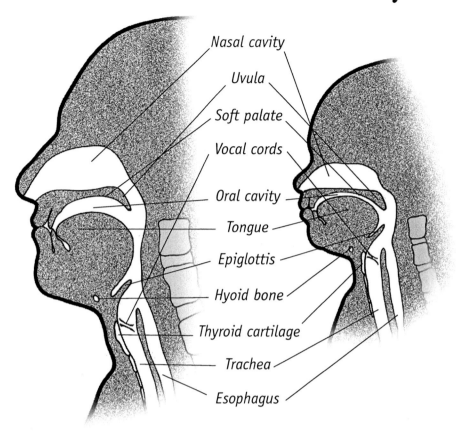

Nasal cavity
Uvula
Soft palate
Vocal cords
Oral cavity
Tongue
Epiglottis
Hyoid bone
Thyroid cartilage
Trachea
Esophagus

Comments and Instructions:

_____
_____
_____
_____
_____
_____
_____
_____
_____
_____
_____
_____
_____
_____
_____

One-Way Speaking Valve

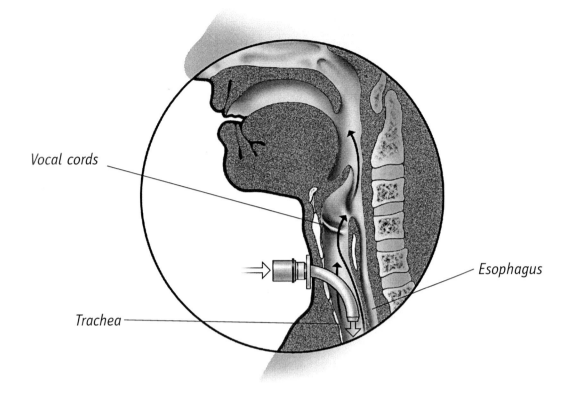

Vocal cords

Esophagus

Trachea

Comments and Instructions:

_____
_____
_____
_____
_____
_____
_____
_____
_____
_____
_____
_____
_____
_____
_____
_____

Stages of Swallowing

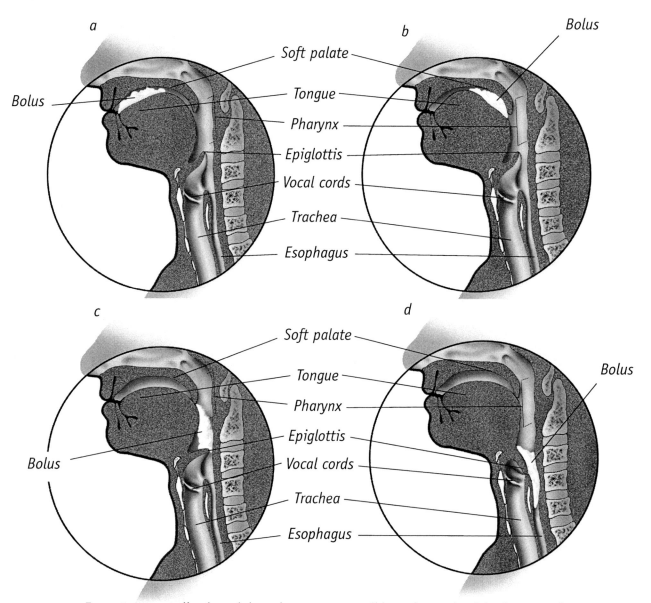

Four stages swallowing: (a) oral preparatory; (b) oral transit; (c) pharyngeal; (d) cervical-esophageal.

Comments and Instructions:

_____

_____

_____

_____

_____

Aspiration with a Tracheostomy Tube

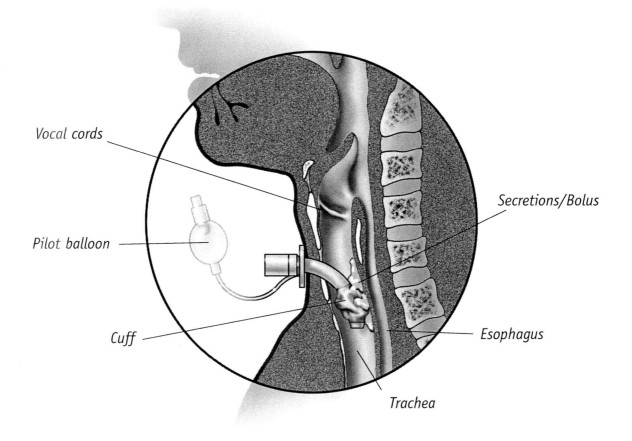

Vocal cords

Pilot balloon

Cuff

Secretions/Bolus

Esophagus

Trachea

Comments and Instructions:

_____

_____

_____

_____

_____

_____

_____

_____

_____

_____

_____

_____

Short-Term Breathing Tubes

a   *b*

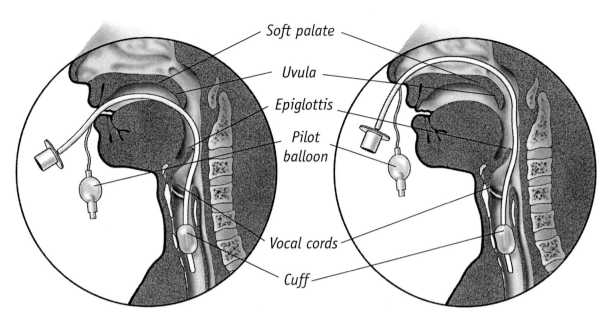

Soft palate • Uvula • Epiglottis • Pilot balloon • Vocal cords • Cuff

(a) Oral Endotracheal Tube Placement and (b) Nasal Endotracheal Tube Placement

Comments and Instructions:

_____

_____

_____

_____

_____

_____

_____

_____

_____

_____

_____

_____

_____

_____

_____

Tracheostomy Tubes and Ventilator Dependence in Adults and Children—VanDahm and Sparks-Walsh

Talking Tracheostomy Tube

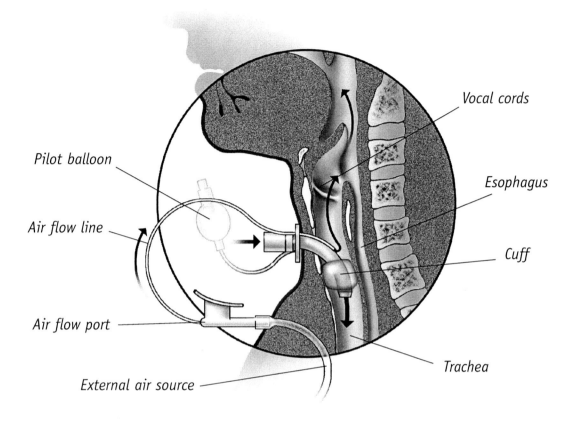

Pilot balloon

Air flow line

Air flow port

External air source

Vocal cords

Esophagus

Cuff

Trachea

Comments and Instructions:

_____
_____
_____
_____
_____
_____
_____
_____
_____
_____
_____
_____
_____
_____
_____
_____

Complications of Overinflated Tracheostomy Tube Cuff

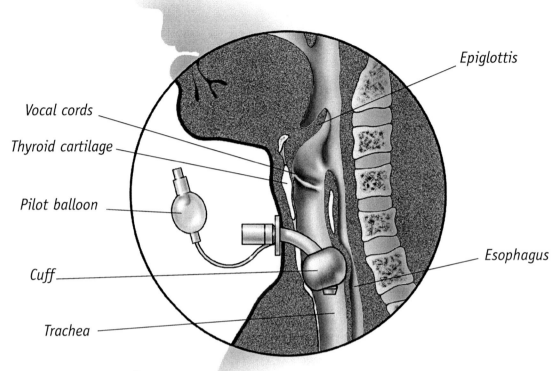

Vocal cords

Thyroid cartilage

Pilot balloon

Cuff

Trachea

Epiglottis

Esophagus

Comments and Instructions:

_____

_____

_____

_____

_____

_____

_____

_____

_____

_____

_____

_____

_____

_____

_____

Glossary

A

AAC: *See* augmentative and alternative communication.

abduction: To move away from the medial plane of the body; for example, opening of the vocal folds.

ABG draw (arterial blood gas draw): A procedure in which a small amount of blood is taken from an artery (usually in the wrist) and analyzed for the concentrations of oxygen and carbon dioxide, pH level and bicarbonate level to assess the adequacy of ventilation and oxygenation.

acidosis: An excessive level of carbon dioxide in the blood, resulting from an accumulation of an acid or the loss of a base. (Respiratory acidosis is the result of excessive retention of carbon dioxide.) It is indicated by a blood pH below 7.35.

adduction: to move toward the medial plane of the body; for example, closing of the vocal folds.

alkalosis: A decreased level of carbon dioxide in the blood, resulting from a deficiency in an acid or the loss of a base (for example, respiratory alkalosis is the result of hyperventilation). It is indicated by a blood pH above 7.45.

alveolus (pl. alveoli): A small hollow or pit; the terminus of the bronchioles in the lungs where oxygen and carbon dioxide are exchanged with the bloodstream.

anterior-posterior transit (*also* A-P transit): *See* oral transit phase.

Apgar score: A rating system used to measure an infant's stability at one, five and ten minutes after birth. The infant's appearance, pulse, respiration, grimacing and activity are rated from zero to two points, for a maximum overall score of ten.

apnea: Temporary absence of spontaneous respiration.

artificial nose: *See* heat-moisture exchange device.

aspiration: The entrance of oral or gastric contents into the larynx beyond the level of the vocal cords. *See also* silent aspiration.

aspiration pneumonia: Acute inflammation of the lungs caused by the inhalation of oral or gastric contents into the lungs; a significant risk for people with dysphagia.

assist-control ventilator (AC): Mode of ventilation that has a preset rate but also assists patient with spontaneous breaths by providing the tidal volume on patient-initiated breaths.

atelectasis: Abnormal condition characterized by partial or total collapse of the alveoli of the lung, preventing the efficient respiratory exchange of oxygen and carbon dioxide.

augmentative and alternative communication (AAC): Any mode of communication other than speech; AAC may be used to supplement or replace oral communication.

B

barotraumas: Injury to the alveoli commonly caused by artificially forcing excessive amounts of air into the lungs via a ventilator.

belly breathing: An atypical breathing pattern characterized by stomach distention with every breath.

bifurcation: Branching; commonly used to describe the point where the trachea divides into the left and right bronchi leading to the lungs (approximately at the level of the fifth thoracic vertebra).

BiPAP (Bilevel Positive Airway Pressure): Often confused with ventilation, it is a non-invasive means of improving ventilation through a continuous rate of inspiratory and expiratory pressures.

bolus: A soft mass of masticated food or collected liquid.

BPM (breaths per minute): A measure of respiratory rate. *See* respiratory rate.

breath stacking: Over-ventilation of the lungs that can occur when a ventilator is not set to accommodate the patient's spontaneous breathing efforts (that is, a patient's breath is stacked on a ventilator breath); results in barotrauma or hyperventilation.

bronchioles: Thin, fine-walled extensions of the bronchus that lead to the alveoli in the lungs.

bronchus (pl. bronchi): Each of the two primary divisions (right and left) of the trachea leading to the lungs.

button (*also* cap, cork, plug): A device that occludes the hub of a tracheostomy tube, allowing the person to breathe normally through the nose or mouth; used in breathing trials when weaning a patient from a tracheostomy tube.

C

cannula (also referred to as the outer cannula): The main shaft of the tracheostomy tube that keeps the stoma open and maintains a patent airway. *See also* inner cannula.

cap (*also* button, cork, plug): *See* button.

cardiac output: The amount of blood circulated by the heart.

carina: A keel-shaped structure; the carina is located at the bifurcation of the trachea into the right and left bronchi and is the area that elicits a cough reflex when stimulated.

cervical-esophageal phase: The final stage of swallowing, in which gravity and peristalsis (rhythmic muscle contractions of the esophagus) propel the bolus through the upper esophageal sphincter into the esophagus and toward the stomach.

chemoreceptors: Sensory nerve cells, triggered by changes in the chemical environment surrounding them, that signal the respiratory center in the brain to increase or decrease ventilation.

cilium (pl. cilia): A small hair-like process found in the nasal passages and lungs. The wave-like motion of the cilium carries mucus, dust, and foreign materials to the pharynx to be expelled.

circulation: The movement of blood throughout the vessels of the body to supply nutrients and carry off waste products.

CMV: *See* controlled mechanical ventilation.

controlled mechanical ventilation (*also* CMV): A mode of ventilation in which the ventilator provides complete ventilator support, with no accommodation for spontaneous breathing by the patient.

cork (*also* button, cap, plug): *See* button.

CPAP (Continuous Positive Airway Pressure): An amount of air pressure provided by a ventilator during spontaneous respiration to overcome the work of breathing through the ventilator tubing and to prevent atelectasis.

cricopharyngeus muscle (*also* upper esophageal sphincter or UES): The superior pharyngeal constrictor muscle. At rest, it is in a closed position; it opens during the normal swallowing process to allow the bolus to pass into the esophagus.

cuff: A soft, inflatable ring around the cannula of some tracheostomy tubes that occludes the trachea, preventing air from passing around the tube.

D

decannulation: Removal of a tracheostomy tube.

diaphoresis: The secretion of sweat, especially the profuse secretions associated with elevated body temperature, physical exertion, exposure to heat, or mental or emotional stress.

diaphoretic: A condition of increased sweating.

diffusion: A component of respiration in which oxygen is dispersed from the alveoli into the bloodstream.

distribution: A component of respiration in which air is moved to the alveoli most effective at gas exchange.

duodenum: The superior section of the small intestines, leading from the stomach to the jejunum.

duotube: A short-term feeding tube inserted through the nose and down the esophagus to the duodenum (the start of the small intestines); used to promote or provide alternative nutrition.

dysphagia: Disorder of swallowing.

E

effortful breathing: An atypical breathing pattern in which every breath appears to be a challenge.

emesis: The act of vomiting.

endoscope: An instrument for visually examining the inside of a tract or hollow organ of the body.

endotracheal tube (*also* **ET tube or ETT**): A short-term artificial airway inserted through the nose or mouth and extending to the trachea.

epiglottic inversion: The action of the epiglottis to cover the larynx during swallowing to protect the airway.

ET tube: *See* endotracheal tube.

ETT: *See* endotracheal tube.

expiration: The act of exhaling air from the lungs.

extubation: The process of removing a tube, such as a breathing tube, from an orifice or cavity of the body.

F

false vocal folds: The ventricular folds beneath the epiglottis and above the true vocal folds.

faucial pillars: Pharyngopalatine (posterior) and glossopalatine (anterior) arches in the posterior oral cavity that separate it from the pharyngeal cavity.

FEES®: *See* fiberoptic endoscopic evaluation of swallowing.

fenestration: Containing holes; describes a tracheostomy tube that has a hole or holes in the posterior wall of the cannula.

fiberoptic endoscopic evaluation of swallowing (FEES®): A procedure in which a flexible nasoendoscope is passed through the nasal cavity to permit observation of the pharynx before and after swallowing.

FiO$_2$: *See* fraction of inspired oxygen.

fistula: An abnormal opening caused by injury, disease or congenital defect. *See also* tracheoesophageal fistula.

flange (*also* **neck plate**): A protruding rim, edge or collar around a tracheostomy tube that sits flush against the stoma. Identifying information about the tracheotomy tube (that is, size, presence/absence of cuff or fenestrations) is located here.

fraction of inspired oxygen (FiO₂): The percentage of oxygen contained in the air a person inhales. The FiO_2 of room air is 21%, and a maximum of 100% FiO_2 can be delivered via ventilator.

G

G-tube: *See* percutaneous endoscopic gastrostomy tube.

gastric-to-jejunum tube (G-J tube): A long-term feeding tube inserted through the abdomen into the stomach and then fed into the small intestines.

gastroesophageal reflux: The movement of stomach contents back into the esophagus.

gastroesophageal reflux disease (GERD): A chronic condition in which stomach contents flow up into the esophagus, causing discomfort and potentially erosion of the esophagus.

GERD: *See* gastroesophageal reflux disease.

glottal incompetence: Inability to completely adduct the vocal folds or close the glottis.

glottis: The opening between the vocal folds.

granuloma: A mass of inflamed tissue.

guppy breathing: An atypical breathing pattern characterized by a wide open mouth and the appearance of gasping for air.

H

heat-moisture exchange device (HME): A device that attaches to the hub of a tracheostomy tube for filtering and humidifying inhaled air.

HME: *See* heat-moisture exchange device.

hub: The proximal end of a cannula or endotracheal tube to which a ventilator (or in tracheostomy tubes, a speaking valve) can be attached.

hyperventilation: A condition that occurs when the volume or distribution of air is greater than the metabolic needs of the body.

hypoventilation: A condition that occurs when volume or distribution of air is not adequate for the metabolic needs of the body.

hypoxemia: Insufficient oxygen in the arterial blood.

hypoxia: Insufficient oxygen at the cellular level.

I

I:E ratio: *See* inspiratory-to-expiratory ratio.

in-line: The use of a secondary device while maintaining connection with mechanical ventilation (such as a speaking valve or sterile suctioning unit).

inner cannula: A part of the tracheostomy tube inserted into the outer cannula.

inspiration: The act of drawing air into the lungs.

inspiratory-to-expiratory ratio (*also* **I:E ratio**): Indicates ratio of time of inspiration to expiration. The normal adult I:E ratio is 1 second inspiration: 2 seconds expiration; infants and children have a shorter inspiratory time of .3–.7 seconds but the expiratory cycle is also shortened proportionately, maintaining an I:E ratio of 1:2.

intercostal muscles: Muscles that couple the ribs together and function as secondary ventilatory muscles.

intrauterine growth retardation (IUGR): An abnormal process in which development and maturation of a fetus stops or slows significantly.

intubation: The process of inserting a tube into an organ or body passage; for example, inserting a breathing tube through the nose (nasal intubation) or mouth (oral intubation) or into the trachea (tracheostomy).

IUGR: *See* intrauterine growth retardation.

J

jejunum: The section of the small intestines between the duodenum and the ileum; a common site for feeding tube placement.

jejunum tube (J-tube): A long-term feeding tube extending into the jejunum through a surgical incision in the abdomen.

K

KUB: An x-ray of the kidneys, ureter and bladder used to verify correct placement of a duotube in the duodenum.

L

laryngeal webbing: An abnormal growth of tissue in the larynx that partially occludes the glottis; may be congenital or due to trauma (a complication of long-term intubation with an endotracheal tube).

laryngoscopy: A procedure in which a fiberoptic scope (laryngoscope) is passed through the nose or mouth in order to observe the action of the vocal folds from above.

leak speech: Phonation accomplished by allowing air to pass around a partially deflated cuff.

Luer valve: A spring-loaded valve on the end of a pilot balloon that prevents air from escaping out of the balloon and allowing the cuff to deflate.

lumen: The channel within a structure of the body, such as the trachea or esophagus.

M

manometer: An instrument that measures the pressure of a fluid; used to measure the pressure in a tracheostomy cuff to ensure adequate inflation.

manual resuscitation bag: A bag attached to a face mask or artificial airway hub that, when squeezed, forces air into the lungs.

MBS: *See* modified barium swallow.

Mendelsohn maneuver: A compensatory technique to assist in laryngeal elevation. It requires the individual to swallow while maintaining an elevated laryngeal position with laryngeal muscles for several seconds prior to releasing.

minimal breathing: An atypical breathing pattern in which little breath flow can be felt from either the mouth or nose.

modified barium swallow (MBS, *also* **videofluoroscopic swallow study, VFSS):** A radiographic procedure in which a patient swallows a barium-impregnated bolus and its transit through the oral and pharyngeal stages is tracked on a video monitor to evaluate swallowing function.

modified Evan's blue dye test: An informal method of checking for aspiration in tracheostomized patients. The patient is given a blue-dyed bolus, and if blue dye is later found in tracheal secretions, aspiration is occurring.

mottling: A spider web–like network of veins apparent just below the surface of the skin, which can occur during episodes of respiratory distress.

N

nasal turbinates: Curved processes that form the nasal passages; they are coated with mucosa that serve to warm, cleanse and humidify inhaled air.

nasogastric tube (NGT): Larger in diameter than a duotube, this short-term feeding tube is inserted through the nose into the stomach. Used to promote or provide alternative nutrition; sometimes hooked to low-wall suction to assist in gastric emptying.

neck breathing: An atypical breathing pattern in which accessory muscles of the neck and shoulders contract visibly during inhalation.

neck plate: *See* flange.

necrosis: Tissue or cell death caused by disease or injury.

negative pressure ventilator: *See* ventilator.

neuromuscular: Relating to or affecting both nerves and muscles.

NGT: *See* nasogastric tube.

NPO: Nothing by mouth; indicates a patient who is entirely dependent on nonoral feedings; from Latin: *non per os*.

O

obturator: Something that blocks a passage or canal; an obturator is placed inside a tracheostomy tube as a guide during intubation and is removed immediately to allow air to flow through the tube.

oral preparatory phase: The initial phase of a swallow in which food is presented to the oral cavity and masticated, or formed into a cohesive bolus.

oral transit phase: The process during swallowing by which a cohesive bolus is propelled posteriorly by the tongue to the pharynx.

P

paradoxical breathing: An atypical breathing pattern characterized by the chest rising as the stomach falls and vice versa.

patency: The state of being open or unblocked.

peak inspiratory pressure (PIP): The highest level of pressure achieved during inspiration; measured in cm H_2O.

PEEP (positive end-expiratory pressure): A small amount of pressure maintained by a ventilator in the lungs at the end of a breath to prevent collapse of the alveoli (atelectasis). Normal PEEP value is 2–5 cm H_2O.

PEG tube: *See* percutaneous endoscopic gastrostomy tube.

penetration: The entrance of oral or gastric contents into the larynx without passing below the level of the vocal cords.

percutaneous: Passed through the skin.

percutaneous endoscopic gastrostomy tube (*also* PEG tube or G-tube): A long-term feeding tube surgically inserted into the stomach through the abdomen.

perfusion: The component of the respiration cycle in which blood is passed through the vessels of the lungs to be oxygenated.

pharyngeal phase: The second stage of swallowing, in which food enters the pharynx and the larynx elevates and moves forward, causing epiglottic inversion.

pilot balloon: A small inflatable sac descending from the flange on cuffed tracheostomy tubes; acts as an indication of cuff status (that is, inflated or deflated).

PIP: *See* peak inspiratory pressure.

plug: *See* button.

PMV: Passy-Muir Speaking Valve.

PO: By mouth; refers to a patient who is able to take nutrition orally; from Latin: *per os.*

positive end-expiratory pressure: *See* PEEP.

positive pressure ventilator: *See* ventilator.

pressure inflation: Spontaneous inflation of a deflated tracheostomy tube cuff over time; characteristic of the Bivona Fome-Cuf®.

pressure support: Extra assistance given by a ventilator to a spontaneous breath to compensate for breathing through the length of ventilator tubing.

pulse oximetry: A non-invasive procedure for measuring the level of oxygen in the arterial blood using a pulse oximeter, an instrument that uses light absorption to estimate the level of hemoglobin (and hence oxygenation) in the blood.

pyriform sinuses: Depressions on either side of the larynx, superior to the upper esophageal sphincter.

R

rate: Refers to the number of breaths per minute delivered to a patient by a ventilator.

reflux: Flowing backwards or ebbing (*see also* gastroesophageal reflux).

residual volume: The amount of air remaining in the lungs at the end of a maximal expiration.

respiration: The process of oxygen and carbon dioxide exchange within the lungs and bodily tissues.

respiratory compromise: A condition that occurs over time in which the body only partially compensates for underlying anatomic or physiologic changes, resulting in inadequate ventilation.

respiratory distress: An acute episode of respiratory insufficiency accompanied by atypical physical and behavioral changes in breathing patterns (including drop in O_2 saturation levels, complaints of dizziness, decreased responsiveness, flaring of the nares).

respiratory failure: A condition that occurs when the exchange of oxygen and carbon dioxide between alveoli and pulmonary capillaries is inadequate and requires intervention in the form of ventilator support.

respiratory rate: The number of breaths per minute (BPM). Normal respiratory rate for infants is 60–80 bpm, for children is 30–40 bpm and for adults is 12-20 bpm.

room air: Refers to normal environmental air, which contains 21 percent oxygen, as contrasted with oxygen-enriched air that may be given to a person who is unable to maintain adequate oxygenation of the blood.

S

sensitivity: In the context of mechanical ventilation, the amount of negative pressure an individual must generate in order to trigger the inspiratory cycle of the ventilator.

serial dilation: A tracheotomy procedure in which a series of dilators is used to create a stoma for the insertion of a tracheostomy tube; the procedure is less traumatic than traditional tracheotomy and allows for more exact sizing of the stoma.

silent aspiration: The entrance of oral or gastric contents into the larynx beyond the level of the vocal cords, without any accompanying behavioral signs (such as coughing, choking).

SIMV: *See* synchronized intermittent mechanical ventilation.

speaking valve: A one-way valve attached to the hub of a tracheostomy tube. This valve allows air to be inhaled through the tracheostomy tube and redirects exhaled air through the larynx, past the vocal cords and out the patient's nose or mouth, making speech possible.

stenosis (pl. stenoses): An abnormal constriction or narrowing of a passage; this may occur in the trachea or bronchi.

stoma: An artificial opening, such as is created by a tracheotomy.

stretch receptors: Specialized sensory nerve endings in the smooth muscles of the airway that assist with the mediation and regulation of inspiration and exhalation.

surfactant: A lipoprotein substance secreted by the alveolar cells of the lungs; it maintains the stability of lung tissue by reducing the surface tension of fluids coating the lungs, preventing the lungs from collapsing and promoting the exchange of oxygen and carbon dioxide with the blood.

synchronized intermittent mechanical ventilation (SIMV): A mode of mechanical ventilation set to coordinate a preset number of mechanical breaths with spontaneous patient breaths. This setting is used to prevent breath stacking (*see* breath stacking).

T

TEF: *See* tracheoesophageal fistula.

tidal volume (*also* **TV or V_t):** The amount of air moved into and out of the respiratory tract during each breathing cycle.

Total parenteral nutrition (TPN): A means of receiving nutrition intravenously rather than through the digestive tract.

TPN: *See* total parenteral nutrition.

tracheoesophageal fistula (TEF): Cell death and erosion of the wall separating the trachea and esophagus, creating an opening between the two tubes. This is one possible complication of a cuffed tracheostomy tube.

tracheomalacia: Softening of tracheal cartilage; prone to collapse. May also be caused by excessive pressure from a cuffed endotracheal tube.

tracheostoma (*see also* **stoma):** The opening created in the trachea during a tracheotomy.

tracheostomy: An opening created in the trachea below the level of the larynx for the purpose of assisting with respiration.

tracheostomy tube: A specialized tube inserted through a tracheostomy and into the trachea.

tracheotomy: Procedure of creating a tracheostomy, or opening into the trachea, in order to gain access to the lower airway.

TV: *See* tidal volume.

U

UES (upper esophageal sphincter): *See* cricopharyngeus muscle.

Upper Esophageal Sphincter: *See* cricopharyngeus muscle.

V

vallecula (pl. valleculae): Any groove, depression or furrow, particularly the ones located between the epiglottis and the root of the tongue.

ventilation: The cyclical circulation and exchange of air into and out of the lungs.

ventilator: A mechanical device that pumps air into and out of the lungs. Positive pressure ventilators, the most common type, operate by forcing air into the lungs. Negative pressure ventilators create a vacuum around the chest, causing air to rush into the lungs (an example is the iron lung).

VFSS: *See* modified barium swallow.

videofluorographic swallow study: *See* modified barium swallow.

videofluoroscopy: The use of videofluorographic techniques to evaluate swallowing. *See* modified barium swallow.

V_t: *See* tidal volume.

W

wean: The process of gradually withdrawing a person from something on which he or she has become dependent (for example, a ventilator or tracheostomy tube).

Bibliography

American Association of Critical-Care Nurses. *Care of the Mechanically Ventilated Patient: Protocols for Practice.* Aliso Viejo, CA: AACN, 1998.

American Speech-Language-Hearing Association (ASHA). Position statement and guideline for the use of voice prostheses in tracheotomized persons with or without ventilator dependence. *Asha*, vol. 35 (Suppl. 10): 17–20 (1993). www.asha.org

American Speech-Language-Hearing Association (ASHA). Scope of practice in speech-language pathology. *Asha*, vol. 38, Spring (Suppl. 16): 16–20 (1996).

Arvedson, J. C., and Brodsky, L. (Eds.) *Pediatric Swallowing and Feeding: Assessment and Management.* San Diego, CA: Singular Publishing Group, 1993.

Campbell, D. Developing competencies in trach and vent care. *ADVANCE for Speech-Language Pathologists and Audiologists* (July 19, 1999): 7–9.

Carrau, R. L., and Murry, T. (Eds.) *Comprehensive Management of Swallowing Disorders.* San Diego, CA: Singular Publishing Group, 1999.

Dettelbach, M. A., Gross, R. D., Mahlmann, J., and Eibling, D. E. Effect of the Passy-Muir valve on aspiration in patients with tracheostomy. *Head & Neck*, vol. 17, no. 4: 297–300 (1995).

Dikeman, K. J., and Kazandjian, M. S. *Communication and Swallowing Management of Tracheostomized and Ventilator-Dependent Adults.* San Diego, CA: Singular Publishing Group, 1995.

Dikengil, A. T., Morganstern, S., Smith, M. C., and Thut, M. C. *Family Articles about Traumatic Brain Injury.* San Antonio, TX: Therapy Skill Builders, 1994.

Engleman, S. G. Early intervention with the Passy-Muir Speaking Valve: Neonates to adolescents. Presentation at American Speech-Language-Hearing Association Convention, San Antonio, TX, November 1998.

Fornataro-Clerici, L., and Roop, T.A. *Clinical Management of Adults Requiring Tracheostomy Tubes and Ventilators.* Gaylord, MI: Northern Speech Services, 1997.

Frey, J. A., and Wood, S. Weaning from mechanical ventilation augmented by the Passy-Muir speaking valve. Abstract form from American Lung Association and American Thoracic Society 1991 International Conference, Anaheim, CA, May 1991.

Golper, L. A. C. *Sourcebook for Medical Speech Pathology.* San Diego: Singular, 1994.

Gordon, V. Effectiveness of speaking-cuffed tracheostomy tube in patients with neuro-muscular diseases. *Critical Care Medicine,* vol. 12, no. 7: 615–616 (1984).

Groher, M. E. (Ed.). *Dysphagia: Diagnosis and Management* (2nd ed.). Stoneham, MA: Butterworth-Heinemann, 1992.

Hoit, J. D. Speak to me. *International Ventilator Users Network News,* vol. 12, no. 3: 3–6 (Fall 1998).

Hoit, J.D. Speak to me...better. *International Ventilator Users Network News*, vol. 12, no. 4: 3-6 (1997).

Hoit, J. D., and Banzett, R. B. Simple adjustments can improve ventilator-supported speech. *American Journal of Speech-Language Pathology*, vol. 6, no. 1, 87–96 (February 1997).

Hoit, J. D., Banzett, R. B., Brown, R., and Loring, S. H. Speech breathing in individuals with cervical spinal cord injury. *Journal of Speech and Hearing Research*, vol. 33: 798–807 (December 1990).

Hoit, J. D., Shea, S. A., and Banzett, R. B. Speech production during mechanical ventilation in tracheostomized individuals. *Journal of Speech and Hearing Research*, vol 37: 53–63 (February 1994).

Iskowitz, M. Intensive intervention for fragile children. *ADVANCE for Speech-Language Pathologists and Audiologists* (April 19, 1999): 7–9.

Iskowitz, M. Intubating the infant: Prolonged ventilation leads to swallowing problems in preemies. *ADVANCE for Speech-Language Pathologists and Audiologists* (July 19, 1999): 10–11.

Kaslon, K. W., and Stein, R. E. Chronic pediatric tracheotomy: Assessment and implications for habilitation of voice, speech and language in young children. *International Journal of Pediatric Otorhinolaryngology*, vol. 9: 165–71 (1985).

Kinsey, G. C., Murray, M. J., Swenson, S. J., and Miles, J. M. Glucose content of tracheal aspirates: Implications for the detection of tube feeding aspiration. *Critical Care Medicine*, vol. 22: 1557–1562 (October 1994).

Klein, M. D., and Delaney, D. A. *Feeding and Nutrition for the Child with Special Needs.* San Antonio, TX: Therapy Skill Builders (1994).

Lichtmann, S. W., Birnbaum, I. L., Sanfilippo, M. R., Pellicone, J. T., Damon, W. J., and King, M. L. Effect of a tracheostomy speaking valve on secretions, arterial oxygenation and olfaction: A quantitative evaluation. *Journal of Speech and Hearing Research*, vol. 38: 549–555 (June 1995).

Manzano, J., Lubillo, S., Henriquez, D., Martin, J., Perex, M., and Wilson, D. Verbal communication of ventilator-dependent patients. *Critical Care Medicine*, vol. 21, no. 4: 512–517 (1993).

Mason, M. Communication approaches for tracheostomized and ventilator dependent patients. American Speech-Language-Hearing Association Invitational Exhibit, 1989.

McPherson, Steven P. *Respiratory Equipment.* 5th ed. St. Louis: Mosby–Year Book, 1995.

Mitsuda, P. M., Baarslag-Benson, R. Hazel, K., and Therriault, T. M. Augmentative communication in intensive and acute care unit settings. In Yorkston, K. M. (Ed.), *Augmentative Communication in the Medical Setting*, pp. 5–57. San Antonio, TX: Communication Skill Builders, 1992.

Murray, K. A., and Brzozowski, L. E. Swallowing in patients with tracheotomies. *AACN Clinical Issues: Advanced Practice in Acute and Critical Care*, vol. 9, no. 3 (August 1998).

Oliver, P. E., Forcht, S., and Lawrence, D. G. Prolonged ventilation effects on feeding and swallowing in premature infants. *Infant-Toddler Intervention: The Transdisciplinary Journal*, vol. 8, no. 3: 211–225 (1998).

Parker, S. C., Intihar, D. M., and Ciardella, A. D. Tracheostomy weaning after head injury. *ADVANCE for Managers of Respiratory Care*, vol. 3, no. 3: 15-16, 38 (April 1994).

Passy, V., Baydur, A., Prentice, W., Darnell-Nell, R. Passy-Muir Tracheostomy Speaking Valve on ventilator dependent patients. *Laryngoscope*, vol. 103: 653–665 (1993).

Passy-Muir Speaking Valves: Effective assessment and treatment strategies to enhance patient outcomes. Irvine: Passy-Muir, Inc., 1999.

Scanlan, C. L., Spearman, C. B., and Sheldon, R. I. *EGAN's Fundamentals of Respiratory Care.* 6th ed. St. Louis: Mosby–Year Book, 1995.

Sengstack, P., and Begley, E. Treating patients with trach tubes in acute care. *ADVANCE for Speech-Language Pathologists and Audiologists*, vol. 9, no. 29: 12–13 (July 19, 1999).

Singer, L. T., Kercsmar, C., Legris, G., Orlowski, J. P., Hill, B. P., and Doershuk, C. Developmental sequelae of long-term infant tracheostomy. *Developmental Medicine and Child Neurology*, vol. 31: 224–230 (1989).

Solomon, B. Swallowing considerations in pediatric medically fragile conditions. Presentation at American Speech-Language-Hearing Association Convention, San Antonio, TX, November 1998.

Spaulding Rehabilitation Hospital, Speech Pathology Department. *Tracheostomy/Ventilator Dependent Clinical Management Program Manual.* Spaulding, NY: Spaulding Rehabilitation Hospital, 1998.

Thomas, P., and Tharp, L. Beyond subacute care: Addressing the special needs of medically fragile children. *ADVANCE for Speech-Language Pathologists and Audiologists,* vol. 9, no. 29: 14-15 (July 19, 1999).

Washington, S., and Martinez, E., Jr. Medical implications in the field of speech-language pathology. Presentation at Medical Speech-Language Pathology Conference, Arizona Speech-Language-Hearing Association Phoenix, AZ, 2000.

Index

AAC devices, 56-57
ABG, 27, 73, 102
AC, 106. *See also* assist-controlled ventilation
acidosis, 27-28
adduction, 74, 119-120
alarms, 105-110
    actions to take, 105, 107
    guidelines for, 107
    settings for use with speaking valve, 112-113
    triggered by use of a speaking valve, 107-108
    types of, 107-110
alkalosis, 28
alveoli, 6, 8, 9-10, 97, 98, 101, 102, 105, 109
    alveolar collapse, 105
amyotrophic lateral sclerosis, 21
anterior-posterior transit, 81
antibiotic-resistant staphylococcus aureus, 128
Apgar score, 14-17, 135
apnea, 21, 98, 108
    alarm for, 100, 108
artificial airway, 5, 53, 98. *See also* intubation
artificial nose. *See* heat–moisture-exchange device
aspiration, 5, 18, 23, 46, 58, 60, 61, 62, 82, 86, 87,
    88, 94, 118, 121
    delayed aspiration, 84
    testing for, 87-91, 92
    with infants, 81
aspiration pneumonia, 17, 79, 95
assist-controlled ventilation, 103. *See also* ventilation
    modes
atelectasis, 101
augmentative and alternative communication, 34, 55-
    56. *See also* AAC devices
barotraumas, 98, 103, 116
belly breathing, 25
bifurcation, 5
bilevel continuous positive airway pressure, 98, 101-
    102
BiPAP. *See* bilevel continuous positive airway pressure
Bivona Aire-Cuf®, 63
Bivona Fome-Cuf®, 41, 58, 61, 67, 111-112
Bivona Talk Trach, 58

bolus, 80, 81, 82, 84, 85, 86, 91, 117, 118, 148, 149
bpm, 25, 100, 103, 106, 135
breath stacking, 103, 104, 116
bronchi. *See* bronchus
bronchioles, 6
bronchus, 5, 126
button, 42
cannula, 36-37, 38, 62, 66, 68, 91, 123
    cuffed versus cuffless, 46-47
    fenestrated versus unfenestrated, 48
    inner cannula, 37, 38, 45, 48, 58, 62, 66, 67-68, 91
    pediatric versus adult sizes, 49-50
    silicone versus metal, 48
    single versus double, 45
    talking versus non-talking, 51
cardiac output, 10, 98
carina, 5
cervical auscultation, 92
cervical-esophageal phase, 79, 80, 81
chemoreceptors, 7
cilia, 3
circulation, 9, 10
CMV. *See* controlled mechanical ventilation
communication, 53-77
    nonvocal options, 55-57
    vocal options, 57-77
    with an endotracheal tube, 55
congenital diagnosis, 21
continuous positive airway pressure, 101-102, 104,
    105, 108
    low CPAP alarm, 109-110
controlled mechanical ventilation, 102-103, 106. *See*
    also ventilation modes
cork. *See* button
CPAP. *See* continuous positive airway pressure
cricopharyngeus, 81
cuff, 16, 32, 38-39, 44, 53, 54, 57, 58, 60-61, 67, 69,
    83, 111, 130
    as protection from aspirated material, 86
    deflation, 94, 111, 112, 115
        to allow phonation, 116
    effect on swallowing, 84-86, 117

impeding laryngeal movement, 83
impingement into the esophagus by, 83
inflating, 32, 38-39
leaking around, 108, 110
misconceptions about, 117
overinflated, 84-85
syringe for inflating and deflating, 130
tolerance of, 87
underinflated, 86
vocal cord function with, 83
decannulation, 95
DHT. *See* nasogastric tube
diaphoresis, 72
dietitian, 20
diffusion, 6, 9, 10. *See also* respiration
distribution, 6, 9-10. *See also* respiration
Dobhoff Tube. *See* nasogastric tube
duodenum, 22, 23
duotube. *See* nasogastric tube
dysphagia, 20, 79-95, 117
in infants, 121
therapy candidates, 117-118
effortful breathing, 25
emesis, 23
endoscope. *See* fiberoptic endoscopic evaluation of swallowing
endotracheal tube, 31, 44, 51, 60, 84, 126, 150. *See also* tracheostomy tube; intubation
adapter for, 66
communicating with, 53, 57
components of, 44
damage from, 60
placement of, 32-34, 54, 150
swallowing with, 84
epiglottic inversion, 81, 82, 83, 94
epiglottis, 10, 11, 32, 79, 80, 81
esophagus, 10
ET tube. *See* endotracheal tube
expiration, 3, 7, 8, 101, 118, 136
extubation, 57, 60, 65
false vocal folds, 53, 79
faucial pillars, 81
FEES®. *See* fiberoptic endoscopic evaluation of swallowing
fenestration, 36, 45, 47, 48, 66, 67. *See also* tracheostomy tube
fiberoptic endoscopic evaluation of swallowing (FEES®), 92, 93, 117-118
FiO$_2$. *See* fraction of inspired oxygen
fistula, 39, 84, 85, 87, 94, 117
flange, 37, 46
fraction of inspired oxygen, 101, 112
G tube. *See* percutaneous endoscopic gastrostomy tube

G-J tube. *See* gastric to jejunum tube
gastric function, 22
gastric to jejunum tube, 23
gastroenterologist, 22
gastroesophageal reflux disease, 23
GERD. *See* gastroesophageal reflux disease
GI specialist. *See* gastroenterologist
glottic closure, 83
glottal incompetence, 33
glottis, 32, 34, 62
glucose strip testing, 91
granuloma, 33, 48
guppy breathing, 25
heat–moisture-exchange device, 43
HME. *See* heat-moisture exchange device
hub, 38, 62, 113
attaching to speaking valve, 62, 65, 66, 68, 113
hyoid bone, 10
hyperventilation, 103, 104
hypoxemia, 33
hypoxia, 89
I:E ratio. *See* inspiratory-to-expiratory ratio
in-line, 64, 66, 68, 98, 101, 107-112, 115-121
in-line suctioning, 126
infectious disease, 128
inner cannula, 123
training patients to remove, 123
inspiration, 3, 6, 7, 8, 64, 101, 106, 118, 136
inspiratory-to-expiratory ratio, 101, 116
intercostal muscles, 6, 7, 8, 72
intrathoracic pressure, 104
intrauterine growth retardation, 14
intubation, 12, 15, 31-34, 101
complications with tracheal, 101
long-term, 34
long-term for children, 12
nasal, 31-32
oral, 31-32
placing a tracheostomy tube, 34-35
short-term, 31-32
using a bronchoscope for, 32
using a laryngoscope for, 32
IUGR. *See* intrauterine growth retardation
J tube. *See* jejunum tube
jejunum tube, 23
Kistner Valve, 62, 65
KUB procedure, 22
laryngeal webbing, 33
laryngeal/pharyngeal sensation, 117
laryngoscopy, 21, 74
larynx, 11, 117
leak speech, 16, 57, 61
Lou Gehrig's disease, 21

Luer valve, 38-39
lumen, 73
manometer, 39
manual resuscitation bag, 32, 33, 107, 109
MBS. *See* modified barium swallow study
mechanical ventilation, 19, 27, 28, 48, 58, 97-121.
    See also controlled mechanical ventilation
        adjustments for speaking valve, 112
        alarms for. See alarms
        infants and children with, 119-121
        placement of speaking valve with, 113
        reading display on, 100-101
        swallowing while on, 117-118
            with infants, 121
        terminology, 100-102
        types of, 98-100
        vocal communication with, 110-111
            candidacy for speaking valve, 111-112
        weaning from, 100, 102, 104, 111
Mendelsohn maneuver, 94
methicillin-resistant staphylococcus aureus, 128
minimal breathing, 25
modified barium swallow study, 18, 85, 88, 92, 117-
    118. *See also* videofluorographic swallow study
modified Evan's blue dye test, 87-90, 92, 117-118,
    121, 128, 131
Montgomery* Speaking Valve, 62, 63
mottling, 76, 120
nasal cavity, 10
nasal pillows, 102
nasal turbinates, 3, 4
nasogastric tube, 22-23
neck plate. *See* flange
neurologist, 19
NGT. *See* nasogastric tube
NPO, 34, 88
nutrition, 21-24
        intravenous, 22
            total parenteral nutrition, 22
        tube feeding, 22-23
obturator, 41-42
occupational therapist (OT), 19
Omni-flex, 98, 110
oral cavity, 10
oral hygiene, 127
oral preparatory phase, 79-81
oral transit phase, 79-81
otolaryngologist (ENT), 19
oxygenation, 101, 105
paradoxical breathing, 25
Passy-Muir Speaking Valve, 61, 62, 64, 66, 94, 102,
    110, 112, 130
        infant with, 119

used with a ventilator, 113, 115
patency, 5, 21, 36, 60, 124-127, 129
PC. *See* pressure control
PCP. *See* primary care physician
peak inspiratory pressure, 101, 108, 112, 115, 120, 121
    alarm, 108
PEEP. *See* positive end-expiratory pressure
PEG. *See* percutaneous endoscopic gastrostomy tube
penetration, 62, 82, 83
percutaneous, 34-35
percutaneous endoscopic gastrostomy tube, 23
perfusion, 9, 10
pharyngeal phase, 79-81
physiatrist, 18
physical medicine and rehabilitation (PM&R) special-
    ist, 18
physical therapist (PT), 20
Pilling Weck Improved Jackson tracheostomy tube, 66
pilot balloon, 35, 38-41, 44, 46, 47, 54, 58, 84, 85,
    86, 145, 149, 151, 152
PIP. *See* peak inspiratory pressure
PMV. *See* Passy-Muir speaking valve
Portex, 63
Portex Trach Talk, 58
positive end-expiratory pressure, 101, 104, 109, 112,
    115, 116
        low PEEP alarm, 109
positive pressure ventilator, 116
pressure control, 105. *See also* ventilation modes
pressure inflation, 41
pressure support ventilation, 100, 104, 105, 106, 108.
    See also ventilation modes
primary care physician, 18
PS. *See* pressure support ventilation
pulmonologist, 18, 97
pulse oximeter, 26, 27, 130
pyriform sinuses, 81
reflux, 23
registered nurse, 19
residual volume, 7
respiration, 3-12, 15, 24-25, 43, 82, 100
        anatomy and physiology of, 3-12
        differences between adult and pediatric, 10-11
        during nippling in an infant, 82
        five stages of, 9-10
        mechanical, 103. *See also* mechanical ventilation
        musculature of, 6-7
        rate for adults, 100
        rate for children, 100
        regulatory function of the brain on, 7-8
        respiratory rate, 25
            atypical, 25
            typical, 25

respiratory status, 24
retaining moisture, 42-43
spontaneous, 103
traumas that interfere with, 20-21
respiratory failure, 120
warning signs, 120
respiratory infection, 128
respiratory therapist, 19, 32, 39, 87, 88, 89, 91, 92, 97, 107, 108, 109, 111, 112, 117, 118, 120, 123
secretion management, 112, 124-127
clearing the airway, 124-126
in-line (or closed) suctioning, 126
oral suctioning, 127
sterile suctioning, 125, 129
supplies for, 130
using a nasal trumpet, 126
sensitivity, 101
serial dilation, 34-35
Shikani-French valve, 62, 65
Shiley® Phonate Speaking Valve, 62, 63
silent aspiration, 92-93
silicone tubes, 48
SIMV. See synchronized intermittent mandatory ventilation
soft palate, 10
speaking valves, 12, 15, 16, 18, 25, 27, 28, 38, 41, 51, 57, 61-77, 87, 92-93, 94, 101, 102, 111-112, 115-116, 124, 130
alarms, 107-110
alternatives to, 116
candidacy for, 67-68
care of, 124
closed-position, 64
criteria for use of, 111-112
difficulties with, 73
during suctioning, 126
fatigue with use of, 64
for metal tracheostomy tubes, 65
helping children adjust to, 76
in-line with a ventilator, 110
one-way, 61, 94
open position, 64, 94
placement, 113
precaution against, 68
protocol for clinical trials of, 69-71
respiratory distress from, 71-72
with a mechanical ventilator, 61
with a metal tube, 48
with infants and children, 73, 111, 119-121
speech-language pathologist (SLP), 20
stenosis, 19, 59, 60, 119

stoma, 58, 68, 95, 129
stretch receptors, 7, 8
subglottic pressure, 82, 83, 111, 117
normalizing, 111
swallowing, 79-95
in infants, 81-82
influence of a tracheostomy tube on, 82-84
phases of normal, 79-81
safety and efficiency with a tracheostomy tube, 93-95
with a tracheostomy cuff, 84-86
swallowing assessment, 87, 117-118, 130
swallowing disorders. See dysphagia
synchronized intermittent mandatory ventilation, 104, 106. See also ventilation modes
talking tracheostomy tube, 57-61, 151
thorax, 12, 103
limiting positive pressure in, 105, 116
thyroid cartilage, 10
tidal volume, 100, 102, 104, 105, 106, 108, 109, 112, 115, 118, 120, 121
to increase, 104, 105, 108, 109
tongue, 10
TPN. See nutrition
trachea, 10, 12
tracheoesophageal fistula, 85, 117. See also fistula
tracheomalacia, 60, 119-120
tracheostoma, 19, 34, 35, 36, 88, 89, 123. See also stoma
tracheostomy, 57
collar, 43
long-term, 57
tracheostomy tube, 34-38, 42, 53, 79, 113, 123, 145. See also cuff; hub
as distinguished from laryngectomy tube, 68
aspiration with, 82, 149
button, 42
cannula, 36-37
cap. See button
care and hygiene, 123-124, 129
dysphagia in users of, 79
fenestrated, 67, 116
hub, 38
humidification, 42-43
neck plate. See flange
obturator for, 41
pilot balloon, 38-39
placement, 34-35, 145
plug. See button
safe swallowing with, 93
types of, 45-51

ventilation alternative to, 98
vocal communication with, 53
tracheotomy, 19, 31, 34-35
percutaneous, 35
Tucker Valve, 62, 66
UES. *See* upper esophageal sphincter
upper esophageal sphincter, 81
uvula, 10, 11
valleculae, 81
vancomycin-resistant enterococci, 128
velum, 118
ventilation, 7, 9-10, 21, 84, 91
in infants, 12
ventilation modes, 102-105
ventilator. *See* mechanical ventilation
VFSS. *See* videofluorographic swallow study
videofluorographic swallow study, 92-93. *See also* modified barium swallow study
videofluoroscopy. *See* videofluorographic swallow study
vocal cords, 10
weaning, 17, 18, 19, 24, 102, 104, 105, 110

About the Authors

Kelly VanDahm is a speech-language pathologist at Select Specialty Hospital in Phoenix, AZ, working with neonates through geriatric patients who have complex medical needs. She received her bachelor's degree in Communication Disorders from Calvin College in Grand Rapids, Michigan, and her master's degree in Speech Pathology from Arizona State University. Kelly also guest lectures at both Arizona State and Northern Arizona Universities and was awarded a Teaching and Learning Effectiveness Grant from Northern Arizona University. She has presented at the Arizona Speech-Language-Hearing Association annual convention and is a member of the Dysphagia and Medical Speech Pathology Committees of the Arizona Speech-Language-Hearing Association. Kelly and her husband, Joel, live in Tempe, AZ with their son, Caden. They enjoy traveling, camping and creative design projects.

Sally Sparks-Walsh is a speech-language pathologist at the Carl T. Hayden Veterans Affairs Medical Center in Phoenix, AZ. She received her bachelor's and master's degrees from Arizona State University. A member of the Association of VA Speech-Language Pathologists, she also has served as chair of the Dysphagia and Medical Speech-Language Pathology Committees of the Arizona Speech-Language-Hearing Association. Currently she is a legislative councilor for the American Speech-Language-Hearing Association, representing Arizona, and is a member of the Executive Board of the Arizona Speech-Language-Hearing Association. Sally has presented at the Arizona Speech-Language-Hearing Association annual convention on the topics of voice disorders, tracheostomy, ventilators and the National Outcomes Measurement System (NOMS). She also has been an invited speaker at the Arizona State University Department of Speech and Hearing Science. Sally is also involved in development of a CD-ROM for dysphagia with the Veterans Administration. Sally and her husband, Kevin, live in Mesa, Arizona. They enjoy traveling, home renovations and the theater.